30-DAY

whole foods cookbook
and meal plan

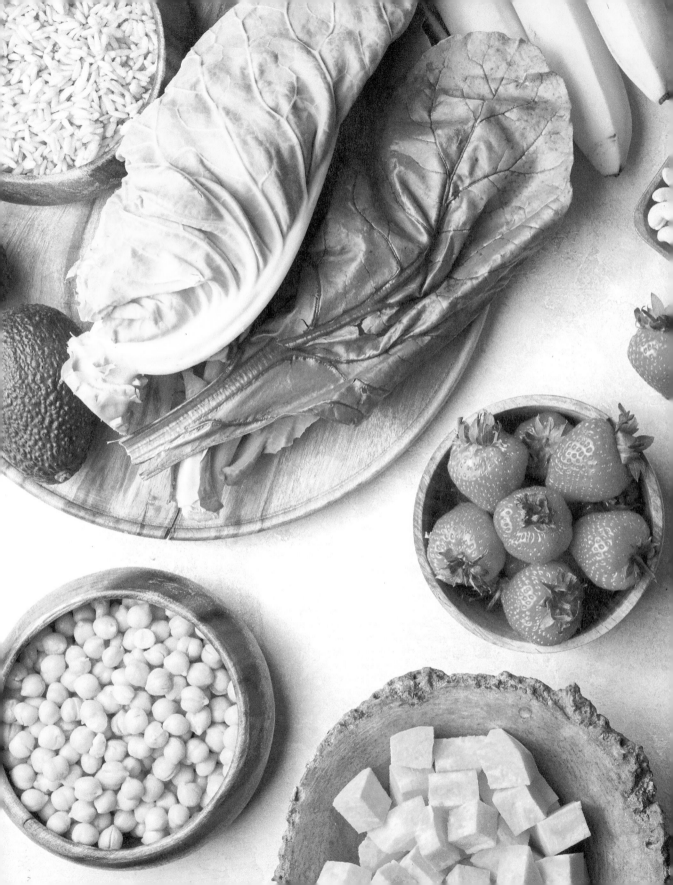

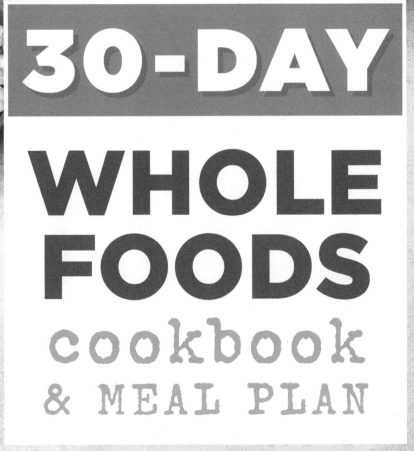

30-DAY

WHOLE FOODS

cookbook
& MEAL PLAN

ELIMINATE PROCESSED FOODS AND REVITALIZE YOUR HEALTH

LORI NEDESCU MS, RD, CSSD

Photography by Darren Muir

ROCKRIDGE PRESS

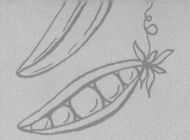

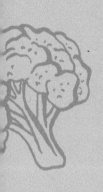

Interior Designer: Lauren Smith
Cover Designer: Katy Brown
Photo Art Director: Karen Beard
Editor: Vanessa Ta
Production Editor: Erum Khan
Photography © Darren Muir, 2018; Food Styling by Yolanda Muir
Illustration © Del_Mar/istock

ISBN: Print 978-1-64152-211-3 | eBook 978-1-64152-212-0

intended for anyone looking to create
a whole, healthy lifestyle by eating
whole, healthy foods.

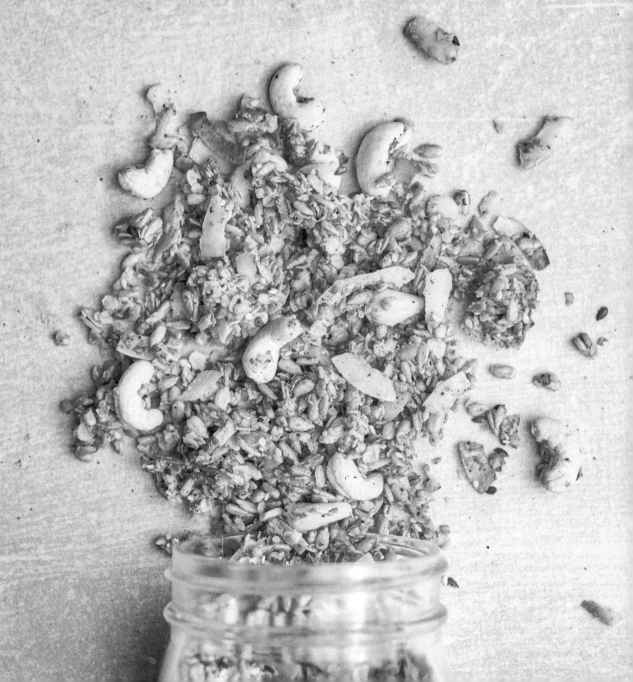

contents

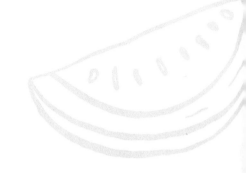

PART THREE: RECIPES

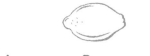

introduction

I cannot tell you how pleased I am that you have picked up this book. Just opening the cover is a step toward committing to a healthier lifestyle by adopting a whole food–based eating style. It is no secret that the foods you choose to eat have an impact on your health and well-being. *The 30-Day Whole Foods Cookbook and Meal Plan* will help you achieve peace of mind that your diet is on track to provide good health, satiety, and balance.

As a registered dietitian nutritionist with over six years of education on diet and human nutrition, over 11 years' experience counseling others on how to eat well, and a true passion for being in the kitchen, I've written this book as a summation of my knowledge, enthusiasm, and practice of cooking and eating a whole food–based diet. Before becoming a nutritionist, I struggled with eating well. I was interested in how food related to health and well-being but too often got caught up in catchy headlines, trends, and practices like calorie counting and choosing packaged foods that offered a plethora of health claims on their labels: Low-Fat! Low-Carb! High-Fiber! Added Protein! Sugar-Free! Low-Calorie! I thought I was eating correctly, but my energy was low, cravings were high, and I had frequent skin inflammation, headaches, mood swings, digestive distress, and weight fluctuations. I needed a change. I devoted my professional career and personal outlook to finding a way of eating that would encompass education, desire, and practicality and emphasize feeling good. Once I reduced my intake of packaged, overly processed foods and shifted toward using whole, plant-based ingredients as much as possible, it didn't take long to feel like a new person. This personal journey is why I am so excited to have you on board to follow this meal plan; I am confident it will transform your lifestyle in a similarly positive way.

Due to the serious benefits plant foods can offer in their whole forms, this diet is very plant forward. However, *The 30-Day Whole Foods Cookbook and Meal Plan* is not about restriction. You'll learn to include many new foods and flavor combinations in your daily eating while on this plan. For those not wanting to go completely plant based, high-quality animal ingredients can still be a valuable component to the diet, just in smaller portions for these 30 days.

Living a go-go-go, nonstop life is the current status quo, making the excuse "I'm too busy" no longer acceptable to neglect good eating habits. Actually, being busy and active is all the more reason to adopt this way of eating, because when we fill our bodies with nourishing foods, our minds are better able to be sharp and focused and our bodies have enough energy to complete important tasks. Keep in mind that as with any new venture, changing your diet will require some initial effort and attention, but the benefits make it completely worthwhile. A whole food diet heavy in plants, like the plan laid out in this book, will promote positive health outcomes such as improved mood, boosted energy, reduced risk of chronic disease, and improved digestion as well as better weight management as you practice mindful cooking and consume nutrient-rich foods. This 30-day guide simplifies healthy eating by providing practical advice, structured meal plans, and inspired recipes all presented in easy to understand terms. The benefits you will experience will likely keep you motivated to continue this style of eating even beyond the 30 days.

Eating the diet outlined in this book—whole, plant-forward, and minimally processed foods—has truly transformed my own approach to fueling for a healthy body, sharp mind, and active lifestyle. I'm thrilled that you're about to experience this positive transformation for yourself.

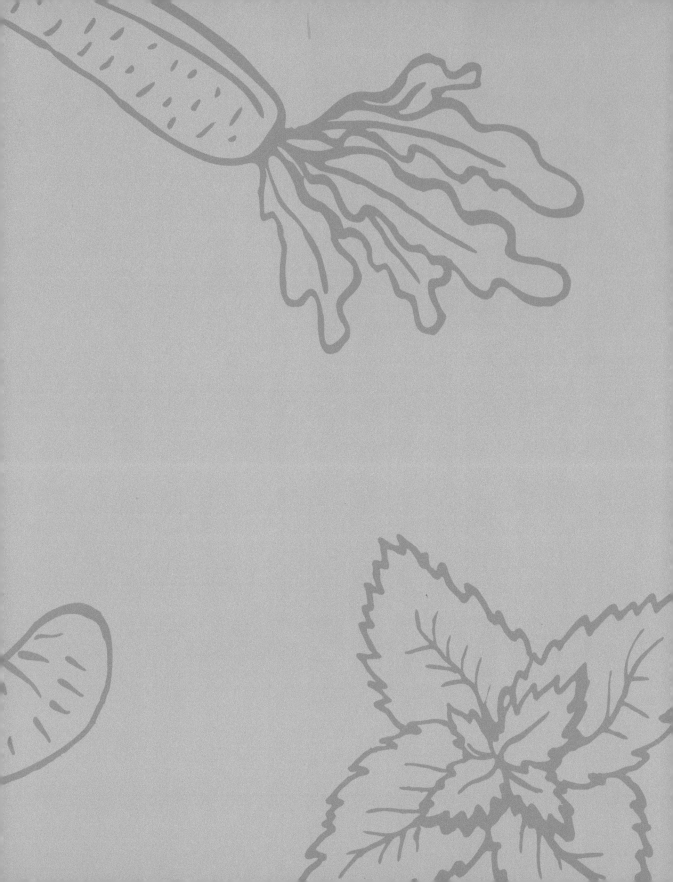

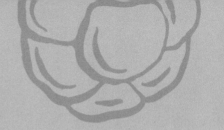

PART ONE

the whole foods diet

There is a seemingly endless amount of confusing information available on the topic of what, when, and how to eat. However, top doctors, researchers, and nutritionists, along with individuals who have made successful nutrition and lifestyle changes, share a common stance: Whole foods are best. Regardless of body type, activity level, or current health status, adopting a diet rich in whole foods will help you achieve your wellness goals.

This section of the book explains in detail what the whole foods diet is, from what constitutes a whole food to which food ingredients should be avoided and those to reach for frequently to the plethora of documented health benefits associated with this style of eating.

After reading this part, you should have the knowledge, confidence, readiness, and excitement to begin your own commitment to 30 days of whole food, plant-based eating.

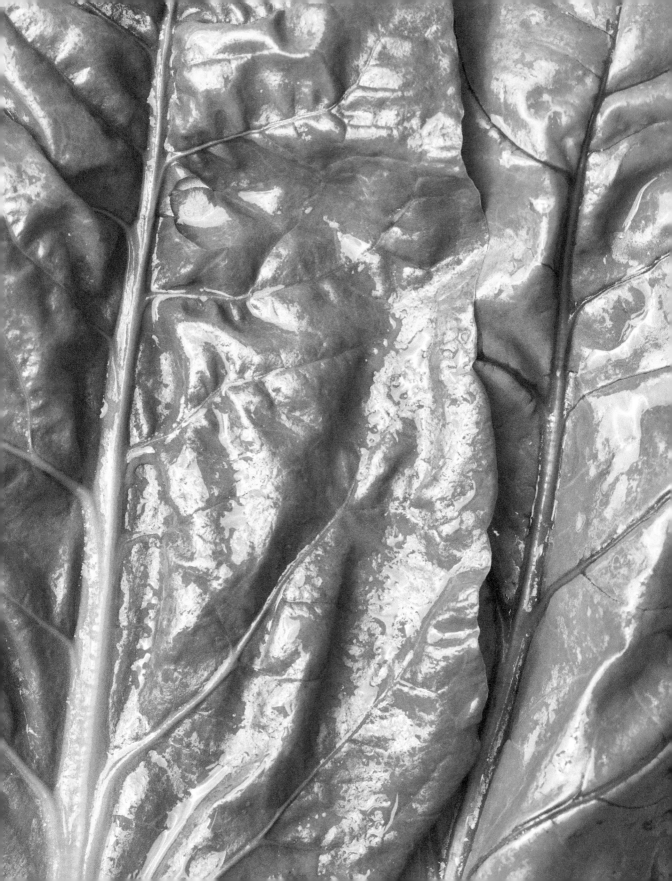

CHAPTER ONE

what is the whole foods diet?

The whole foods diet is an approach to reducing the amount of packaged, processed, and premade foods consumed. By replacing these less nutritious ingredients that make up a large portion of most Americans' diets with nutrient-rich, colorful, filling, and tasty whole ingredients as detailed in this 30-day plan, you'll see improvements in your overall health and energy levels.

In this chapter, the concept of the whole foods diet is explained to create a deeper understanding of the plan. So if you're still scratching your head about what a whole food really is, don't worry. This definition, along with a thorough listing of which foods to choose and which to avoid, is given in the following pages. This chapter will also ignite your enthusiasm to commit to the whole foods diet for the full 30 days by exploring the reasons behind its creation, such as explaining the enticing (and scientifically backed) health improvements you can expect while on the plan.

BENEFITS

Chances are, you're not picking up a diet book just for fun; you're looking for results. While there will be some fun had while following this plan (seriously!), the whole foods diet is designed to get results. There is almost no health- or wellness-related goal that can't be helped by adopting this way of eating. There are so many potential benefits to eating a diet rich in whole foods that it would take a much, much longer book than this one to describe them all, but knowing some of the lifestyle improvements that can take place from eating this way will help motivate your adherence throughout the 30 days, so let's take a peek at a few key potential benefits.

Living longer with good health is a goal we can all get behind. Unfortunately, there are many chronic diseases that work against aging well. The World Health Organization claims that outside of genetic and environmental factors, the food you eat has the largest effect on health outcomes such as high blood pressure, diabetes, mental decline, poor digestion, low bone density, and obesity. Consuming a plant-heavy, minimally processed diet contributes to the decreased risk of many diseases and chronic health conditions. This is exactly the eating style (whole foods, plant heavy, minimally processed) prescribed in this plan, which means that by following the whole foods diet, you'll be making huge improvements to your overall health outcomes.

Like I mentioned earlier, we are all very busy people, so who couldn't benefit from extra hours in their day? I know I could. Sad news: That's impossible. Happy news: Eating whole and minimally processed ingredients contributes to boosted energy levels, meaning you can accomplish more in less time. Having seemingly endless energy stems from your body being able to process food efficiently. The efficiency of this process, known as metabolism, is increased when supplied with balanced macronutrient intake, high levels of micro- and phytonutrients, and appropriate caloric portions consumed at regular intervals.

Bodies can't be energized 24/7, as rest is crucial to good health. Deep sleep regulates hunger levels, replenishes energy levels, and even contributes to muscle synthesis. Most Americans struggle to get the recommended amount of sleep each night, a fact clearly linked to daily food intake. More specifically, diets high in processed foods and sugar and low in fiber contribute to poor sleep habits. This is exactly the type of food intake this diet reduces. Looking forward to high-energy days and restful nights just by eating delicious whole foods seems like a good investment.

Let's face it: Looking good is important to well-being, too. Having a positive self-image is linked to increased confidence, self-worth, and success. Good thing a diet rich in whole foods provides a large variety of antioxidants and anti-inflammatory compounds to increase skin's luminosity, elasticity, and youthfulness. By limiting processed foods, you also limit exposure to additives and preservatives that can cause skin issues such as dulling, redness, breakouts, and dryness.

Oh, did I skip over weight loss? Yes, but on purpose. This diet is primarily intended to improve your health and your eating habits. You will most likely experience weight loss by following this plan due to whole foods filling you up on less calories; however, research shows that dieting with the sole purpose of weight loss is often abandoned. Weight loss on its own just isn't enough of a motivating factor for long-term results. For these 30 days, put weight-loss goals on the back burner, instead keeping track of health and lifestyle improvements that will lead to a stronger relationship with food and behaviors for long-term success.

food & our environment

The whole foods diet is not only good for your personal well-being but also benefits the environment. Animal consumption is expensive, both in what you pay out of pocket and the cost to the environment, which is a very large carbon footprint. It takes extensive resources (land, water, pesticides, fertilizers, feed, labor, and energy) to produce the massive numbers of animals consumed on the Standard American Diet. While going completely vegan has the lowest carbon footprint, it isn't necessary to completely give up eating animals and animal products to make an impact. The Environmental Working Group claims that a family of four who gives up eating steak one meal a week (that's just one out of the 21 meals you consume a week) for an entire year has the same impact on the environment as not driving their car for three months. A claim like that is hard to ignore; we all want to live in a world that is thriving. By relying less heavily on animal products, you will contribute to a more sustainable environment. Choosing animal products that are raised locally (visit your farmers' market), limiting the number of ruminant animals (cattle, sheep) you consume, and including more vegetarian or vegan meals in your weekly menu are all ways to positively impact your body and the environment. The whole food diet in this book recognizes that plant foods (grains, fruits, vegetables, nuts, legumes, and seeds) sustain and promote not only individual health but the health of the world around us as well.

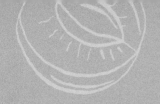

animal products

The 30-day whole foods diet is mainly plant based due to the undeniable nutritional benefits plant foods provide and the fact that most of our diets seriously lack these foods. That doesn't mean that animal foods are bad. Far from it. They provide protein, B12, iron, satiety, and balance. For this reason, animal products are not excluded on the 30-day plan. Animal products include any food that comes directly from a living creature (steak or shrimp) or is derived from one (whey, cheese, butter). When following the whole foods diet, aim, as far as you are able, to choose animal foods that are high-quality, such as those that are grass-fed, pasture-raised, wild, local, sustainable, and minimally processed. For example, eggs from pastured hens, grass-fed beef, and wild salmon are options included on this plan, while deli meats, hot dogs, and fish sticks are not.

Remember that this diet's main goal is to steer you toward eating whole foods. Many animal products tend to be less processed than plant-based meat substitutes. For example, soy crumbles would be a heavily processed, less-optimal alternative to grass-fed organic ground beef. Just as when choosing other foods, animal products should resemble their true state as much as possible (like a sardine or chicken thigh) and be single-ingredient foods even if minimally processed (butter or plain yogurt). The goal is to keep overall animal consumption to around 15 percent of your total dietary intake, leaving plenty of room for plant foods. When adding an animal ingredient to a meal, think of it as a side rather than the main component. However, don't get too caught up in specifics; the goal is to eat mostly plant based, but if you want to eat animal products, choose the best-quality options rather than worry about the exact amount.

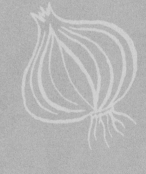

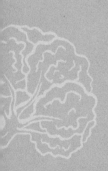

Of course, your individual results will vary based on your starting status and commitment to sticking with the plan for the full 30 days, but you can be confident that simply by following this plan, you will see an improvement in your overall well-being.

Are you motivated and excited to begin the whole foods diet and start seeing results for yourself? I hope so. Of course, to get started, you need to know what this plan is all about.

WHAT IS IT?

In a nutshell, the whole foods diet is a plan to increase the amount of (you guessed it) whole foods that you eat. But there's a little more to it than that. On this plan, for a span of 30 days you'll commit to shopping for, preparing, and consuming a diet that is mostly plant based and that features whole food ingredients with a few supplemental, lightly processed foods. This approach is intended to guide you to better nourishment by increasing awareness, knowledge, and positive habits. The whole foods diet plan will help you be mindful of how your body responds to food, instead of trying to control it. For example, instead of stressing over strict calorie guidelines, learn to recognize when you feel full and when to naturally stop eating.

Diets that restrict or shove habits into a box are difficult to follow and often lead to frustration and abandonment, which is why this plan is very inclusive. The whole foods diet permits supplemental lightly processed foods, and animal products are not off-limits. Whether you need to be gluten-free or wish to eat a Mediterranean, Paleo, or vegan diet, the whole foods diet can be adapted to meet your individual nutrition and lifestyle needs. The only eliminating you'll do is of overly processed, packaged foods. Everything else is on the menu.

what are whole foods?

This plan takes you beyond the "rabbit food" that may come to mind when someone mentions plant-forward, whole food eating and introduces you to a wide range of delicious options. Eating less-processed whole foods can be exciting, fun, colorful, and tasty. As with any new concept or venture, it will take a little work and practice to get the hang of it, but rest assured that the new habits will stick and this way of eating can be easily integrated into your lifestyle. So what is a whole food? The term refers to any food in its original state (or as close to it as possible) with minimal refining, additives, or processing. Whole, less-processed foods are easy to spot in any

can eat

√ **Fruits:** all fresh, frozen, dried, freeze dried, and unsweetened purées

√ **Vegetables:** all fresh, frozen, dried, freeze dried, pickled/fermented, and unsweetened purées

√ **Grains:** amaranth, brown and wild rice, buckwheat, corn, farro, millet, old-fashioned and steel-cut oats, quinoa, and wheat berries

√ **Legumes:** canned, dried, and frozen beans, lentils, and peas

√ **Complete meals:** whole ingredient soups, stews, and grain blends

√ **Nuts and seeds:** all raw/sprouted varieties and plain spreads, and nut/seed butters

√ **Dairy:** organic cottage cheese, kefir, milk, and plain yogurt

√ **Beverages:** coffee, 100 percent fruit or vegetable juice, kombucha, matcha, unsweetened plain nut milks, unsweetened tea, and water

√ **Plant proteins:** edamame, tempeh, and tofu

√ **Animal proteins:** free-range poultry, game meats, grass-fed meats, pastured eggs, uncured sausage, and wild seafood

√ **Fats and oils:** avocado oil, coconut oil, ghee, grass-fed butter, olive oil, and toasted sesame oil

√ **Condiments:** broths, coconut aminos, fresh salsa, hummus, miso, plain mustard, tamari, and vinegars

√ **Supplements:** baobab, cacao, cordyceps, maca, plain protein powders (collagen, hemp, pea, and/or whey), reishi, and spirulina

√ **Herbs and spices:** fresh, dried, and frozen, with no sugar or salt added

√ **Sweeteners:** honey, maple syrup, and molasses

√ **Snack foods:** air-popped popcorn, baked vegetable chips, minimally processed seed crackers, fruit and nut bars, and trail mixes with whole food ingredients only

See, like I promised, there are plenty of items you can still eat. Basically, anything whole, unpackaged, and minimally transformed!

can't eat

X **Fruits:** sugar-added varieties

X **Vegetables:** sauce- and salt-added varieties

X **Grains:** instant oats, packaged pastas and breads, pilafs, premade granola, pre-made pizza crusts, and sugary cereals

X **Legumes:** pre-sauced varieties

X **Complete meals:** boxed, canned, and frozen options, including pizza and burritos

X **Nuts and seeds:** candied varieties, sugar-added nut/seed butters

X **Dairy:** chocolate, flavored yogurts, ice cream, processed cheeses

X **Beverages:** alcohol, fruit-flavored drinks, soda, a sweetened milk, tea, coffee, and water

X **Plant proteins:** processed meat substitutes

X **Animal proteins:** bacon, cured sausages, deli meats, imitation seafood, and pro-cessed meat products

X **Fats and oils:** imitation spreads and sprays, and vegetable oil

X **Condiments:** balsamic glaze, jams, mayonnaise, and premade dressings/sauces

X **Supplements:** sweetened and artificially sweetened blends

X **Herbs and spices:** seasoning mixes and packets

X **Snack foods:** baked goods, candy, chips, fried ingredients, premade bars, pretzels, and trail mixes with candy and coated bits

Simply stay away from items in packages with long ingredient lists that do not resemble a natural whole food. Instead of being overwhelmed by the "can't eat" list, focus on all the good foods you can still include!

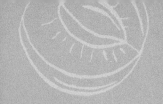

organic vs. conventional

On the whole foods diet, you're advised to choose organic versions of foods as much as your lifestyle allows. For reference, organic ingredients are grown without pesticides, synthetic fertilizers, and genetically modified organisms (GMOs). Ingredients claiming to be organic undergo routine testing to ensure they meet the organic definition. Animal products labeled as organic must not have been given antibiotics or growth hormones. On the flip side, the term "conventional" covers any food item not meeting organic standards, meaning they may contain or have been exposed to synthetic growing materials, pesticides, and GMOs. GMOs are foods that have had their original, organic DNA structure altered to achieve a specific goal, such as a higher edible yield, more uniform shape, increased protein, etc. While this process creates successful crop populations, it is unclear if they promote, or harm, one's health. While the research is inconclusive, common sense says that consuming food altered from its original state is suboptimal. Avoiding GMOs by choosing organic and non-GMO products is a precautionary measure to ensure you're doing everything you can to promote good

health. While the nutrition fact labels for organic and conventional produce might look similar, organic foods contain higher levels of phytonutrients. These compounds include antioxidant and anti-inflammatory compounds that are vital to promoting a healthy body. It might be ideal to eat 100 percent organic ingredients, but it simply isn't realistic for most of us to adopt a completely organic diet due to financial concerns or limited availability. The Environmental Working Group publishes a Dirty Dozen™ and Clean Fifteen™ list each year (see Appendix A, page 181) of produce most and least contaminated by pesticides. These lists will enable you to prioritize your purchases by choosing to buy organic versions of the foods you eat frequently and those on the Dirty Dozen™.

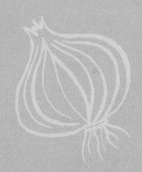

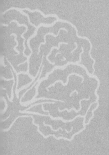

grocery store by simply determining how closely the food item resembles the original food. For example, an apple is a whole food, applesauce is a slightly processed version of apples, and apple toaster pastries are a highly processed version. Choosing the apple would be the best option. Choosing a natural applesauce is a good way to get closer to the real thing. Whole food options go well beyond fruits and vegetables. There are whole and less-processed options in every category (grains, produce, nuts, seeds, meat, and fish) of food group. Buying the most original forms possible will ensure the meals and snacks you create adhere to this new style of eating and promote positive, healthy outcomes. The goal is to fill your cart, kitchen, and therefore plate and body with nutrient-rich, less-processed foods.

Focusing on the larger goal of positive lifestyle changes will help keep you from getting too caught up in the details of what a whole food is or is not. For example, olive oil is processed from the olive fruit, but as a single-ingredient, nutrient-rich product, it counts as a whole food. Honey is another example of a technically processed yet still whole, nutrient-rich food. This book tells you which foods and ingredients are appropriate for this plan and which should be avoided for at least the first 30 days, so don't fret about remembering all this right now, because you can always flip back to these pages for reference.

You might find that the biggest change for you is making meals from scratch instead of buying a premade final product. Be confident that this does get easier with a little practice. The recipes and advice in this book will guide you to cooking new and flavorful foods using simple techniques, keeping things interesting on your 30-day whole food eating adventure.

10 Staple Whole Foods

- Almonds
- Avocados
- Bananas
- Berries
- Brown rice
- Chickpeas
- Eggs
- Leafy greens
- Oats
- Sweet potatoes

what are processed foods?

Processed foods come in many forms; some are quite beneficial and permitted on this diet while others can work to derail all your health ambitions. Some minimal processing simply creates a more convenient product, like ready-to-eat hard-boiled eggs, frozen blueberries, and canned tomatoes. These items can be a great addition to your diet by simplifying the tasks of shopping, preparing, and cooking. Other, more processed foods add a variety of extra ingredients (sugars, preservatives, additives, gums, and fillers) to make a ready-to-eat product that is far from the original form, such as frozen pizza, bologna, and teriyaki sauce. Extra ingredients like high-fructose corn syrup and nitrates in these processed foods have been linked to poor health outcomes, according to the World Health Organization. The stripping away of nutrients—such as the increasing loss of fiber when oats are transformed from steel-cut to old-fashioned to quick-cooking to instant—that occurs in processing reduces the nutritional quality of the food.

Heavily processed items like premade meals, frozen dinners, or boxed side dishes can be the easiest versions of processed foods to spot and avoid, while the minimally processed items can be a bit trickier to see. A simple way to choose the "right" processed foods is to look at the nutrition label. Underneath the nutrition facts panel, you'll find the ingredient list. Check this information for extra ingredients you wouldn't typically expect to find in the food you're holding. For example, frozen broccoli should list only broccoli. If you see sodium, milk proteins, etc., put the bag down and try again. Another example is tomato sauce. There are many versions that list tomatoes as the first ingredient and contain only other vegetables, herbs, and spices. However, there are many more jars that list sugar as the first ingredient, followed by a long list of other items you might not associate with the simple notion of tomato sauce. Use this technique to navigate the aisles, and as time goes on, the selection process will become much easier. This plan focuses on whole foods, but no one expects you to churn your own butter or extract oil from olives, so some healthy, minimally processed foods are included.

10 Processed Foods to Avoid

- Candy/sweets
- Chips/fried snacks
- Cured meats
- Frozen/boxed ready-to-eat meals
- Packaged baked goods/pastries
- Processed cheese slices
- Sauces, spreads & dressings
- Sugary beverages
- Sugary cereal
- White bread/ refined flours

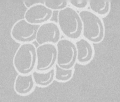

eating out

Following the whole foods diet is a lifestyle approach, meaning there is leniency. You have a busy, active life and your diet should support that, not work against it. Ideally, every meal would be prepared in your own kitchen from high-quality, whole ingredients, but—reality check—life happens. We've all been caught in situations that require grabbing a bite while you're away from home. When you're on the go, traveling, eating at a friend's, having a business lunch, or simply left your super healthy meal sitting on the kitchen counter (it happens), being prepared to handle these situations is part of adapting this diet to your lifestyle.

Keep the principles of this diet (whole foods, plant forward, minimally processed) in mind when making choices of what to eat outside your meal plan recipes. When looking at a restaurant menu, look for straightforward, single-ingredient options and avoid overly descriptive or mixed dishes. For example, a salmon fillet with roasted potatoes and broccoli would be better than lobster mac 'n' cheese with creamed spinach. A vegetable omelet with fruit would be a better option than sausage and biscuits with gravy. Another way to navigate menus is to look for meals similar to what your meal plan suggests. For example, if the meal plan lists Mixed Grilled Vegetables (page 146), look for some form of grilled vegetables on the menu. Remember that you have a say in what you are served, so don't be shy about requesting something not on the menu, such as combining several side items or asking for no bread and sauce on the side. Having to grab food on the go is not a reason to abandon your plan. Stay strong and focused on the big picture of improving your health and eating habits.

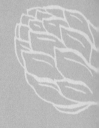

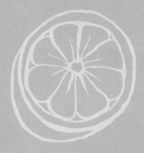

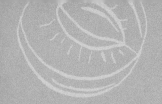

sugar

Simply stated, sugar is a problem in the Standard American Diet (yes, that is abbreviated to SAD). Our processed food supply is loaded with sugar because it is a cheap way for companies to add a likeable flavor to everything from pasta sauce to yogurt to canned soups and even hamburger buns. The addition of sugar creates an addiction-like response in the brain. We like it and we want more of it. Except that the more we eat, the more we crave, and the more we consume, the more our health deteriorates. Sugar consumption has been linked to diabetes, weight gain, depression, and degenerative mental conditions.

During the initial part of the whole foods diet plan, you might experience headaches, fogginess, and intense cravings while your body adjusts to not eating so much sugar, but toward the end of the 30 days, you should be experiencing increased clarity, focus, energy, motivation, and few, if any, cravings.

It doesn't mean you have to never taste sweet again. During this plan, you'll reset your taste buds to not require hyperstimulation from sugary foods in order to be satisfied. You will also learn to taste the sweetness in natural foods like carrots, apples, and corn. Sugar in the form of maple syrup, molasses, and honey are allowed on the whole foods diet because they are in fact whole, single-ingredient, minimally processed foods that contain some nutritional benefits. They are still sugar, though, so you should use them only in small amounts and combined with other nutrient-rich whole foods, especially fiber, which slows the rate at which the sugar is broken down. For example, chopped dates add a burst of sweetness to Moroccan Carrot Salad (page 94), and maple syrup is used to sweeten the Sunflower-Oat Granola (page 76). I promise you, this diet is sweet in all the right ways.

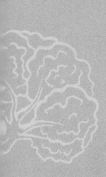

THE WHOLE FOODS DIET BREAKDOWN

The 30-day whole foods diet provides you with a simple plan of what to eat for each meal each day. It includes tasty recipes, shopping guidelines, and meal prep tips. The plan follows a three-meals-a-day structure and gives snack options to keep you fueled all day. How much you consume should be based on your personal needs, activity level, and hunger levels. The word "diet" typically indicates eating less; however, a diet based on whole plant foods (like this one) is nutrient dense compared with the calorie-dense Standard American Diet, meaning you get more food volume for the same calories. Eating mindfully and chewing slowly will help you pay attention to when you are truly satisfied and should stop eating.

While eating this way might come as a change, it should be an exciting one. The recipes aim to break you out of your comfort zone (and nutritional rut) by introducing new flavors, ingredients, and preparations, like using squash ribbons as noodles and cashews to make a creamy, cheesy sauce. When trying new recipes and unfamiliar foods, keep an open mind and remember why you are doing this diet in the first place: your health. Focusing on the benefits you stand to gain—youthful skin, higher energy levels, improved body composition, reduced cravings, deeper sleep, and decreased disease risk—will keep you motivated to move forward day after day.

Trying new foods is crucial to including a greater variety of plant-based nutrition, but there is no need to go overboard. While a few of the recipes might challenge you to break out of your comfort zone, like the Miso-Mushroom Stir-Fry (page 117), others are whole food versions of classic favorites, like the Sloppy Joe Lentil-Stuffed Peppers (page 122).

The whole foods diet meal plan and accompanying recipes follow the plant-forward, whole food, minimally processed foundation, but they allow for plenty of flexibility for individual needs. Remember, learning to make this eating style work for you is important to developing successful long-term habits.

the whole foods diet

In essence, the diet is this: Eat a large amount of whole plant foods, a moderate amount of minimally processed plant foods and animal products, and a scant amount of the rest. That's the secret to eating for optimal well-being. If it seems too simple, well, that's because it is. Whole, single-ingredient plant foods (fruits, vegetables, grains, legumes, nuts, and seeds) should make up the majority of your meals. Supplement with smaller portions of high-quality animal ingredients (sardines, eggs from pastured hens, and grass-fed meat), minimally processed foods (coconut oil, canned tomatoes, whole-grain flours, maple syrup, and vinegars), and limited-ingredient packaged items (bars, soups, sauces with only whole ingredients listed, nut milks without gums and fillers). Anything else should be as minimal as possible. All too often we try to overcomplicate healthy eating with trendy supplements or restrictive plans that just lead us to an unhealthy on/off diet cycle. The whole foods diet will get you back to the simple basics of eating a diet that is nutrient rich, accessible, and adaptable and promotes positive health outcomes.

who can follow this diet?

This diet is appropriate for anyone and everyone. For those in special circumstances, such as pregnant or breastfeeding women, young children, and serious athletes, it is important to adapt the diet to your individual needs. While the foundation remains intact, the amounts and proportions of macronutrients may change. Pay attention to eating until satisfied, your energy levels, and your general health. If you're concerned, contact a dietitian who can adapt this plan more specifically to meet your specific needs.

why 30 days?

If this way of eating is such a golden ticket to health and well-being, why only 30 days? Shouldn't one just always eat like this? Yes! However, adopting new habits and behaviors takes time and some effort. In the beginning, the risk of feeling overwhelmed and abandoning your efforts is high, especially if you think that the diet is "forever." Thirty days is less daunting a time span than "forever." Committing to just 30 days will help you stick with the diet, but there's more to it than just focusing on a short-term goal. Research has shown a new habit takes at least 18 days to form, so this length of time (30 days) will help your new habit become part of your lifestyle. During this period of time, it is crucial to follow the meal plan advice strictly. In the future, you'll be able to adapt it more to your personal needs and preferences, but for this 30-day period, commit to following the plan. By doing so, you'll help reduce your body's cravings for sugary, overprocessed foods. Over the course of the meal plan, living without such foods will become normal, and the initial temptation to reach for unhealthy products will wear off. Think of it as a detox period; you are ridding your body of previously ingested junk and resetting your system to crave healthier options.

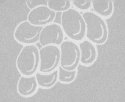

eating with the seasons

When on a plant-based, whole foods diet, the best nutrients and flavor come from choosing foods that are in season. For example, tomatoes taste best in late summer, strawberries in early summer, and most greens are more vibrant in early spring. Have you ever bought a grocery-store tomato in January and been disappointed by the mealy, flavorless taste? Picking foods that are in season will help you truly experience the flavors plants can offer. As a bonus, produce is less expensive in season. During peak harvesting times, there is more supply of the plant than meets demand, which drives the price you pay way down. You get better-quality, better-tasting food and spend less: win-win.

Make seasonal food work for your whole foods diet by learning what grows when in your region, visiting your farmers' market, and learning to make substitutions in your recipes. Kale is a colder-weather green, and the leaves can turn bitter once temperatures rise. If your salad recipe calls for kale but it is June, swap it for arugula, which will give a peppery twist to your salad. Pan roasting fresh cherries with balsamic can make a lovely sauce in July, but in January, opt for frozen cherries because frozen (single-ingredient, additive-free) produce has the peak-season nutrition and flavor locked in. Making these seasonal swaps is an easy way to avoid suffering recipe boredom and try new variations with minimal effort.

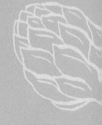

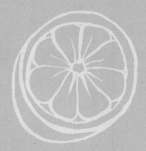

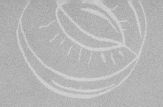

food & mood

Having a bad day? There's a food for that. While "good mood food" sounds too catchy to be real, it is definitely a legitimate concept. The brain relies on nutrients to process information and stay alert, and it houses the center for emotions, stress, anxiety, and mood. Foods rich in DHA, an omega-3 fatty acid found primarily in fish, assist with flexible, healthy cell membranes and normal neuron functioning. Tryptophan is an amino acid found in many grains that leads to serotonin (a natural "feel good" compound) production in the brain. Try having a complex carbohydrate–rich snack like air-popped organic popcorn to improve your sense of happy and calm. Blueberries are also a great choice when you need a mental lift. These richly colored berries are loaded with antioxidants that target cognitive function. Magnesium, a mineral found in leafy greens and seeds, is linked to reducing anxiety.

Improving gut health can also go a long way toward boosting mood. There is a connection between the gut and the brain; even Hippocrates stated that all disease begins in the gut. By eating simple, whole, nutrient-rich foods and decreasing processed, calorie-dense junk ingredients, you can have a stronger mind-gut connection. Probiotics are microorganisms that help good bacteria flourish in the gut, improving digestion and the mind-gut connection. Fermented foods are loaded with probiotics, which is why natural, unsweetened, organic kefirs, yogurts, and aged cheeses are allowed in small amounts after your 30-day "detox" period. To include probiotics during the 30 days, opt for kimchi or sauerkraut.

While you might be tempted to reach for chips or cookies during times of stress or sadness, remember that although these foods may provide temporary relief, they come with lasting negative effects. Choosing whole foods with mood-boosting qualities will leave you blissful now and later.

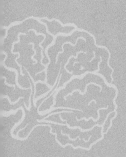

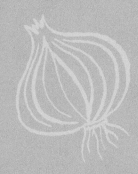

During these 30 days, you won't be eating dairy- and gluten-containing foods. These are not necessarily unhealthy foods, and it will be fine to reintroduce whole food versions once the 30 days are up. However, eliminating them for an extended period, then reintroducing, is a good way to determine how your body feels "on" versus "off." When you add these items back in, pay extra attention to how you feel. If you experience lethargy or fogginess, you might have a sensitivity to a particular food and want to continue a diet free of it.

If you do slip up during these 30 days, don't worry. You're human, and mistakes happen. If you do get off track, here's how to handle it. If the indiscretion is limited to a single event (a piece of cake at a wedding), then shake it off and get right back to the plan. If you become completely derailed for several days, start fresh by thinking through what caused you to abandon the plan and how you can avoid that in the future, then commit to a new 30-day period. Slipups are normal, as changing old habits is a difficult task to truly accomplish. Stay confident that this process is worth it, and don't give up on yourself.

FOOD AS MEDICINE

As you now know, the acronym SAD stands for Standard American Diet, and sadly (pun intended), it's no surprise that it is commonly known as SAD. The way Americans tend to eat—heavy in empty calories, low-quality meats, and fast, overly processed foods—has led us down a path of poor health. Obesity, heart disease, cancer, and diabetes are major health issues that affect the well-being of our country's citizens. The Centers for Disease Control and Prevention (CDC) states that over 35 percent of American adults are obese, which increases the risk of many chronic health issues. Obesity is promoted by low activity levels and high consumption of calorie-dense, nutrient-poor, overly processed food products (exactly the opposite of what the whole foods diet proposes you eat).

Heart disease is one of the leading causes of death in America, and part of what fuels this disease is a lack of fruit and vegetable consumption. A study by Produce for Better Health found that only one in 10 American adults eats the recommended amount of fruit and vegetable servings a day. While there are many types and causes of cancer, there is enough research to suggest that diet plays a role. High consumption of processed meats (cured sausages, luncheon meats) has been linked to certain types of cancer, while consumption of whole plant foods has been shown to decrease risk. Type 2 diabetes is a very serious health condition, yet preventable. The largest risk factor for type 2 diabetes is obesity and obesity-related health concerns, such as high blood pressure, high cholesterol, inactivity, and elevated blood sugar levels. Increased risk of nonalcoholic fatty liver disease, asthma, gestational diabetes, multiple sclerosis, polycystic ovarian syndrome, and depression have all been linked to overconsumption of processed meats.

In all these serious diseases there is evidence that suggests eating a diet rich in produce, fiber, and nutrient-dense and minimally processed foods will greatly lessen your risk. No research suggests a diet high in sugary, nutrient-poor, overly processed foods will help prevent disease or promote health. Almost every researched nutrition intervention calls for increased intake of legumes, vegetables, fruits, nuts, and seeds. It seems like such simple advice, yet we neglect to follow it, perhaps because our taste buds have become too accustomed to the SAD diet.

Not only do these chronic health conditions lead to risk of premature death, they also contribute to high medical costs and a poor quality of life. Quality of life refers to how well you feel and how easily you can do general daily tasks and activities without having shortness of breath, pain, fatigue, or other general suffering.

Connecting the food choices you make with your personal health and quality of life is the first step to improved outcomes.

There are countless stories of people being cured of health issues by focusing on diet. Magazines, TV shows, medical reports, case studies, personal blogs, and social media accounts can be found that highlight how someone transformed their health by changing their diet to a healthier, nutrient-rich one. For example, a young London-based nutritionist was able to drastically reduce psoriasis after reducing sugar intake, a 59-year-old man claims a strict diet of plant shakes reversed his type 2 diabetes, and a 33-year-old woman who battled depression for years ditched her SAD eating style for unprocessed foods and found herself in good spirits. These stories are just a tiny sample of what people experience when making the switch to a plant-forward, whole foods diet. The Forks Over Knives (a plant-forward eating style) website boasts a full page of people claiming to have cured or reduced any number of health issues by improving their diets, and magazines like *Women's Health* have a monthly feature of transformation by focusing on healthier lifestyle behaviors. While these stories are amazing examples of the power of diet and lifestyle, all too often the dietary revolution came after years of suffering, medications, and exhausting other resources with no success.

Even if you aren't at any immediate risk of a chronic health condition and feel that your quality of life is pretty good, you can still benefit from eating the whole foods diet. This diet is meant to do more than decrease disease risk. It promotes

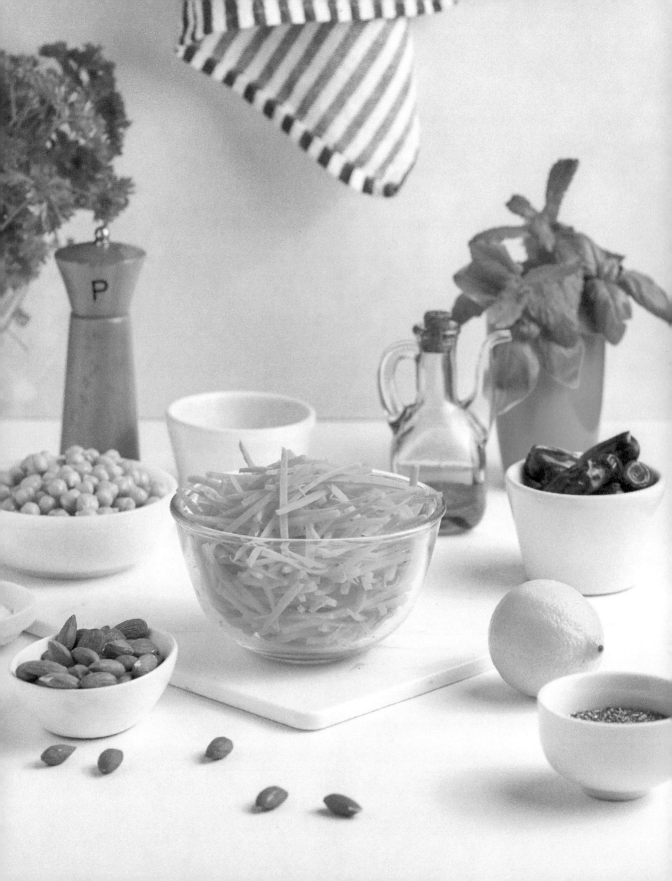

well-being. A dull complexion, mood swings, headaches, grumpy stomach, poor sleep, and feeling lethargic throughout the day are all quality of life issues that can be connected to the foods you consume. They can also all be addressed by following this meal plan. By eliminating overly processed foods, lessening animal food consumption, and focusing on whole plant foods, you can gain vibrancy, focus, and energy and reduce the negative effects of daily stress and inflammation. The diet helps in more ways than merely telling you what to eat; it helps create a more mindful environment for eating by providing tips for shopping, meal prep, simple recipes, meal balance, and structure.

Foods popular on the Standard American Diet create a SAD outlook for our health and well-being, but there are plenty of foods on the whole foods diet that actively promote good health.

health-promoting foods:

Blueberries: Bursting with color and flavor, these little gems are loaded with antioxidants (specifically anthocyanins) that target the breakdown of fat cells and reduce the risk of hypertension and cognitive decline (like poor memory and Alzheimer's disease).

Avocados: These fatty fruits (yes, officially a fruit) are great for promoting satiety, meaning you'll stay fuller for longer, so no cravings or excess snacking. They've also been linked to reducing hypertension and combating oral cancer.

Tomatoes: Lycopene gives tomatoes their rich red hue and also supplies the ability to fight off eye degeneration, hypertension, hyperlipidemia, and even some cancers.

Fatty fish: DHA, a key omega-3 fatty acid supplied almost exclusively by fatty fish varieties (including salmon, mackerel, herring, and cod), is responsible for brain health and fighting depression.

Dark leafy greens: These vegetables provide bulk, filling you up with fiber and nutrients for very few calories. This makes them ideal for weight control. The extensive nutrient profile of vitamins, micronutrients, and phytonutrients make them perfect for promoting an overall strong system.

Eggs: Forget the whites only. Pasture-raised organic egg yolks are great sources of choline, which promotes production of acetylcholine, a neurotransmitter for nerve functions associated with mood, muscle, and memory.

Sweet potatoes: Filling due to the high fiber content, these root vegetables are a great whole food carbohydrate source to load up on. They work to promote a healthy complexion and weight control and might play a role in reversing diabetes and heart disease.

Almonds: A clinical trial has shown that eating almonds increases the availability of vitamin E in the body. This vitamin is a powerful antioxidant that helps combat heart disease, blood sugar, and some cancers and assists in reducing muscle soreness.

Mushrooms: One of the few food sources of vitamin D, mushrooms can help with bone health. Most notable, however, is their ability to boost the immune system's ability to fight off infection and illness.

Beets: The deep red root vegetable contains natural nitrates (not to be confused with the dangerous nitrites in processed meats), which help increase blood flow, helping lower blood pressure and even boosting athletic performance.

Of course, this is just a small sample of some of the heavy hitters. Each and every whole food plays a role in promoting a healthy body and mind in its own individual way.

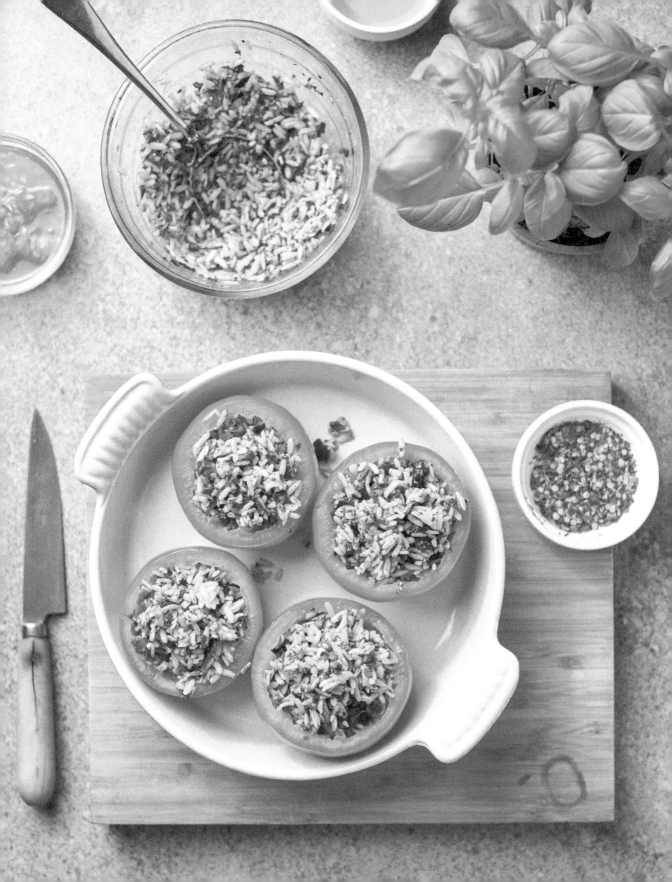

CHAPTER TWO

getting started

By this point, you are well versed in the rationale behind this diet and the health benefits it will bring, and you're probably eager to get started. Before you hit day 1, however, there are some basics to cover to get you prepared for a successful 30 days. Throughout this chapter we'll discuss what to expect to get you mentally prepared and motivated to tackle the diet and reduce any stress or overwhelming thoughts about beginning. We'll also discuss how to prepare your kitchen—refrigerator, freezer, pantry, and equipment—to handle the new style of eating. By the end of this chapter, you should feel excited and ready to embark on this new lifestyle journey.

WHAT TO EXPECT

The good things in life are worth working for. You've probably heard this saying many times before, and it really applies here while you're preparing for the whole foods diet. These 30 days will be demanding; you're going through a big lifestyle shift and changing habits related to what you eat, how you eat, and how you think about food as it affects your body. These first days might not be easy, but they will be worth it. Going into this period with confidence, hope, and a little preparation is key to making it to the end. Whenever you start to feel a little frustrated, remind yourself of the rewards you will reap and your personal goals for making these changes.

The first week is usually the most trying as old, unhealthy habits are abandoned and replaced by new, health-driven ones. To make it easier on yourself during these initial days, schedule more time for shopping, prepping, cooking, and eating as you learn to choose the right foods, meal prep, and make things yourself instead of grabbing premade versions. The first part is the most tedious, but the learning curve isn't steep on this diet, and soon these new tasks will be easy and second nature. As you adapt, the time spent preparing your meals will decrease, giving you more time to enjoy the results. While some results, such as weight loss, lowered blood pressure, and disease prevention, may not be immediately obvious, don't be discouraged. Rest assured the process started the moment you replaced your old habits with the whole foods diet. Focus on the results you will see immediately, like improved mood, energy levels, glowing skin, and better mental focus.

Beyond the time and attention you'll need to invest in the initial days, there are some temporary issues you might experience. Essentially, these 30 days are a detox for your body, ridding it of toxins and poor food choices. The more extreme the difference between your old diet and what is prescribed here, the more intense your period of detox will be. During this time, it is common to go through some withdrawal-like symptoms such as intense cravings, fogginess, and headaches as your body comes off its SAD sugar high. This period is short lived, although admittedly a bit miserable. You can get through this! The stricter you are with your new habits, minimizing "slipups," the faster and more easily you will get through it. To make it easier, reduce time spent in social food situations (meet friends for yoga or a game of pickup basketball instead of happy hour), skip the doughnut-laden break room at work (keep approved snacks at your desk), and if your normal commute takes you past a line of tempting food chains, find a new route (the route to success). Tell your family, roommates, friends, and coworkers that you will be starting the whole foods diet. There's no need to be pushy or attempt to convert those around you; your job is to focus on you. Let them see for themselves the benefits you are reaping, and they'll soon be begging to know your secret. Making those around you aware of your diet goals is a way to take responsibility and commit to your actions. Again, during this time, it is important to stay strong and remind yourself of why you are doing this and the benefits you stand to gain.

In the end, 30 days is a tiny portion of your life that can make a lasting positive impact on your well-being by staying strong and committed to the whole foods diet.

PREPARING YOUR HOME

Preparing yourself mentally is step one. The next step is to prepare your home, mainly the kitchen. If you share a kitchen with others, explain to them what you hope to achieve, then create pantry, refrigerator, and freezer space that will be yours alone. If the kitchen is already yours alone, go on a "kitchen cleanse," tossing out (or donating to a food pantry) all the foods not allowed on the plan—the fewer temptations the better. When poor food choices are not immediately in reach, you are less likely to give in to them. When your kitchen space is cleansed of unhealthy, overly processed foods, you will be able to begin restocking it with the whole, minimally processed, health-promoting foods allowed on this plan.

pantry

Maintaining a well-stocked pantry is crucial for healthy-eating success. These are the foods that will be readily available for your consumption, so make good choices. Without all the boxed and bagged items taking up space, you can use your pantry to support your whole foods diet. While fresh whole foods will take center stage, the pantry items listed will help you create flavorful, balanced meals.

Stock your pantry with the following:

- Broths: bone and vegetable
- Canned fish: salmon, sardines, and tuna
- Canned tomatoes and beans
- Dried beans, lentils, and peas
- Dried fruits
- Dried herbs and spices
- Grains: brown and wild rice, oats, and quinoa
- Honey

- Maple syrup
- Nut and/or seed butters, including tahini
- Oils: avocado, coconut, extra-virgin olive, and toasted sesame
- Popcorn kernels
- Raw nuts and seeds
- Supplements (optional): baobab, cacao powder, collagen powder, cordyceps, hemp or pea proteins, maca, nutritional yeast, reishi, spirulina, turmeric, whey, etc.
- Tamari or coconut aminos
- Unsweetened shredded coconut
- Vinegars: apple cider, and red and white balsamic

refrigerator

This is where most of your approved foods will hang out. These foods are most perishable; keep small amounts on hand and shop frequently for the best-quality products. Use your refrigerated items to create the bulk of your meals, using pantry and freezer ingredients to supplement and enhance the fresh ingredients.

Stock your refrigerator with the following:

- Animal proteins, if using (see list on page 8)
- Fresh, 100 percent fruit and vegetable juices
- Grass-fed butter
- Kombucha
- Mineral water
- Olives
- Pastured eggs
- Plain unsweetened nut milks
- Sauerkraut and pickled vegetables
- Seasonal fruit
- Seasonal vegetables
- Tofu and tempeh

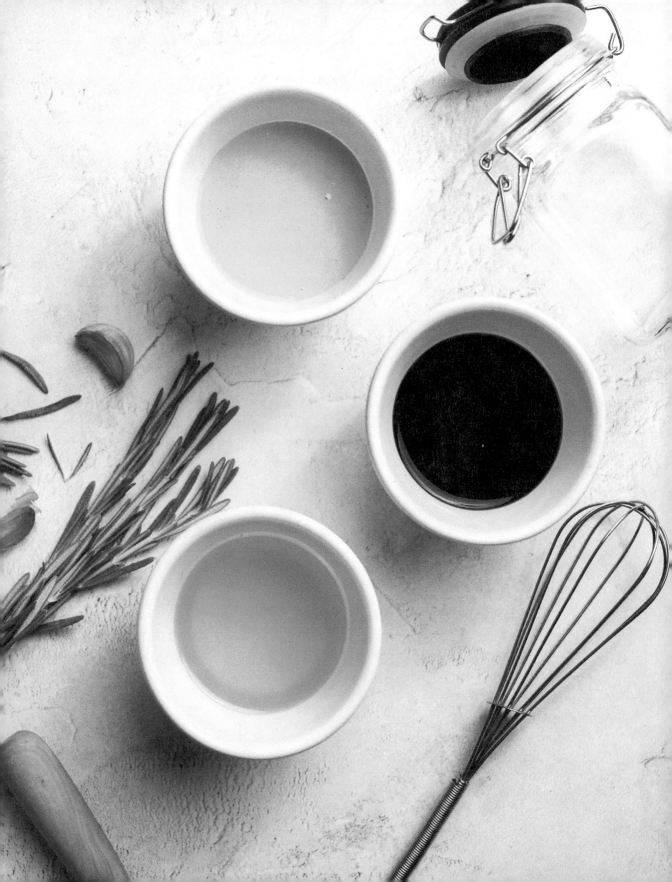

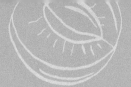

freezer

Frozen foods generally bring to mind heat-and-eat style, overly processed premade meals. Now is your chance to rethink frozen foods. Frozen ingredients are normally frozen as soon as they are caught or harvested, thereby locking in flavor and nutrients and giving you the ability to eat unseasonal ingredients without nutritional sacrifice. A diet of fresh produce and proteins requires frequent trips to the market due to their high perishability. This can be offset by keeping a stock of frozen ingredients, which last much longer, are generally less expensive, and add a welcome bit of convenience. Stock your freezer with harder-to-prep produce, like frozen butternut squash and beets, to make life easier. Pricey fruit like acai, berries, and figs (especially when out of season) and seldomly used specialty items like artichoke hearts or shitake mushrooms are also great freezer picks. For this meal plan, you can use plain, frozen cooked grains, corn, fruit, peas, spinach, and squash. Another great choice for your freezer is individually wrapped meat and fish portions, if you are consuming them. Buying frozen helps save money when making the switch to grass-fed and wild varieties of animal proteins, and the individually packed portions help make just enough, no more and no less. Just as when buying fresh and pantry ingredients, seek out the best-quality frozen items you can.

equipment

Turning whole food ingredients into meals doesn't require a state-of-the-art kitchen setup or a fancy culinary degree. To ease the transition to cooking meals yourself, there are a few kitchen tools you might find helpful. You most likely already have some of these in your kitchen. You might be skeptical of some items at first, but they are sure to become more frequently used than your toaster and microwave once you start making recipes from whole food ingredients.

Good knife and cutting board: Make sure your knife is sharp, as you're going to be doing a lot of chopping, slicing, and dicing in the next 30 days.

Pots and pans: Give them a good clean and move them to an accessible spot in your kitchen. These will also get used plenty over the next 30 days and hopefully beyond that.

Blender/food processor: When making your own dressings, energy bites, soups, and smoothies, you will deeply appreciate having a good blender. Many modern varieties like the Ninja and the Vitamix act as high-powered combination food processors/blenders and are ideal for making smoothies and grinding nuts. While they might be a little pricey, they will be put to constant use in your new way of eating. Think of it as a worthy investment.

Rice cooker/Instant Pot: A rice cooker will make your life easier as the grain does take about 40 minutes to cook on the stovetop. Being able to add rice and water and click a button greatly frees up time for other activities. If you have the means, forgo the rice cooker (which, as the name suggests, is a bit limited in its range) and opt for an Instant Pot, which can assist with speedy pressure cooking of eggs, rice, and even beets.

Spiralizer: This gadget is a type of peeler that creates long ribbons or "noodles" from any vegetable.

Mandoline: This tool helps slice fruits and vegetables into uniform thicknesses. Biting into a raw radish may not sound super appetizing, but adding very thin slices of radish to a meal can change the way you think of the ingredient. A mandoline will introduce produce in a way that is inviting and not overwhelming to your taste buds. It also saves time because instead of laboriously cutting vegetables, you can just "swipe" a vegetable over the blade and be done. When buying this item, pair it with a cut-resistant glove to avoid accidents.

Microplane: Commonly known as a "zester," this little grater will help you add bursts of flavor to your meals. Use it to zest citrus and grate fresh ginger, garlic, or chiles into dishes for natural, whole food taste enhancement.

Milk frother: This handheld, battery-powered mini immersion blender thickens and froths milk and other liquids. You can also use it to add powdered supplements to drinks, like collagen into coffee or turmeric into oat milk.

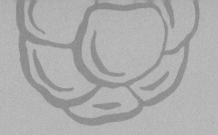

PART TWO

meal plan

You're probably pretty excited to get going at this point, but before you dive into the meal plan, there are some basics to cover. The idea is to follow the plan as given, but making it work for you is more important than obsessing over exact details. Let your schedule and preferences guide you to make any necessary adjustments and tweaks to the plan by swapping meals between days, weeks, and categories. For example, swapping Monday's meals with Thursday's meals is fine, and if you just love Tuesday's lunch, making a big batch to eat all week works, too. You can also eat leftover breakfast as a snack or dinner for lunch. The meal plan repeats recipes to simplify shopping and prep, but there are many additional recipes in chapters 8 through 11 that you can choose from to keep things interesting if you find yourself with extra time and ambition.

The important concept to strictly commit to is using whole foods and lots of plants and forgoing processed ingredients, excess sugar, and large (if not all) animal food portions for these 30 days. You should also stick to eating three balanced meals and one snack per day that are roughly the same portion size, meal to meal, day to day. In other words, no tiny breakfasts and oversize dinners or mindlessly pick- ing at snacks all day; consistency is important. Try to avoid meals

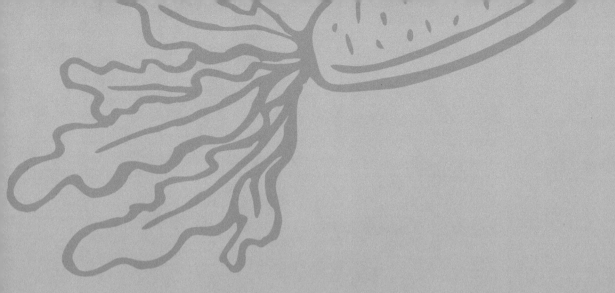

consumed in social settings during this time, as doing so can tempt you into making choices that don't adhere to these guidelines. The meal plan advises batch cooking once a week to reduce the arduous task of cooking three meals a day from scratch by doing some prep work and having key components cooked and ready. During these 30 days, always carry a whole food, plant-based snack for situations where you're hungrier than expected, on the go, or in another situation that could tempt you away from meal plan–approved choices.

Desserts are not included on the meal plan. This is to keep your focus away from treats and sweets and on the important concept of consuming lots of whole, healthy foods and limiting extras during this 30-day period. However, we all need a little occasional indulgence to keep from feeling deprived. Luckily there are plenty of ways to transform whole foods into delicious (and more nutritious) desserts. I've included some of my favorite whole food dessert creations in the recipe section (page 133) to help you learn to make treats that are better for your body and health. These desserts should not be a part of your everyday meal plan but should instead be added occasionally into your 30 days for special occasions and when you really need a treat.

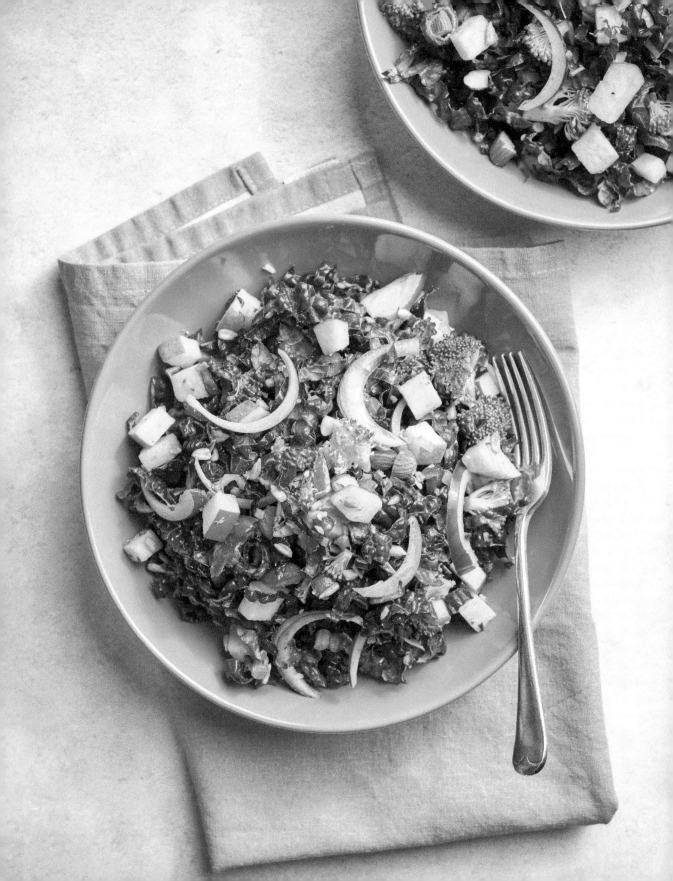

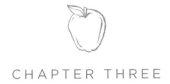

week one

Are you ready? Now that you've read all about the diet and prepared your kitchen, it's finally time to begin. During this first week, you might struggle with devoting the extra time to planning, grocery shopping, food prep, and cooking meals from scratch, but don't get overwhelmed. As stated earlier, this process will get easier each day as you become confident using whole foods, and the benefits are so worth the effort. At the end of this week, you should feel more comfortable with the process. You should also feel excited about cooking and eating whole foods, aware of how much food your body needs, and enjoying increased clarity and energy levels.

OPPOSITE: DATE & ALMOND KALE SALAD, PAGE 123

PREP AHEAD

To make things easier on yourself, try preparing a few things in advance. This way, you will have ingredients ready to toss into meals, saving lots of time and effort. Throughout the weeks, make extra of any recipe you will be using again later in the week to save time and effort. If making extra salads to have later on, keep the dressed and warm parts separate to add over fresh greens at the last minute. For example, this week you will have the Peach & Sweet Potato Salad (page 113) twice. Make double of the peach and sweet potato (warm) part and store that away to reheat and serve over the cool, crisp greens days later. This method will help you with batch cooking and leftover preparation throughout the 30 days.

For week 1, prepare the following items ahead of time:

- Sunflower-Oat Granola (page 76)
- Bird Bread (page 164)
- Coconut Rice (page 155), or plain brown rice
- 2 baked sweet potatoes per person
- Creamy Balsamic Dressing (page 174)
- Honey-Lime Dressing (page 175)
- Almond Oat Milk (page 168)
- Crispy Chickpeas (page 150)

WEEK 1 SHOPPING LIST

Check your pantry, refrigerator, and freezer to see what you already have.

pantry

- Bee pollen
- Chickpeas, canned
- Coconut aminos or tamari
- Coconut milk, canned
- Coconut water
- Coconut, unsweetened shredded
- Fruit, dried: dates and raisins
- Grains: brown rice, oats, and quinoa
- Herbs and spices, dried: Balti seasoning, caraway seeds, cardamom (ground), cayenne pepper (ground), chipotle pepper flakes, cinnamon (ground), cumin (ground), ginger (ground), paprika, poppy seeds, red pepper flakes, and turmeric (ground)
- Nut butter of choice
- Nuts, raw: almonds and cashews

- Oils: avocado, coconut, olive, toasted sesame, and walnut
- Olives
- Psyllium powder
- Seeds: chia, flax, hemp, pumpkin, sesame, and sunflower
- Supplements (optional): collagen powder, nutritional yeast, and/or protein powder
- Sweeteners: honey and maple syrup
- Tahini
- Tomatoes, canned
- Vinegars: apple cider, balsamic, and white balsamic

refrigerator/freezer

- Apples (4)
- Avocados (4)
- Bananas (4)
- Basil (1 bunch)
- Broccoli (1)
- Cabbage, green (1)
- Carrots (1 pound)
- Cilantro (1 bunch)
- Dill (1 bunch)
- Garlic (1 head)
- Ginger (1 knob)
- Kale, lacinato (1 bunch)
- Lemon (2)
- Limes (4)
- Mint (1 bunch)
- Mixed greens (1 large container)
- Nut milk of choice (1 container)
- Onions, sweet (2)
- Onions, red (5)
- Orange (1)
- Orange juice, 100 percent (1 carton)
- Parsley (1 bunch)
- Peaches (8)
- Pepper, jalapeño (1)
- Peppers, red bell (7)
- Pineapple (1)
- Potatoes, sweet (5)
- Rosemary (1 bunch)
- Shallot (1)
- Squash, summer (2 large)
- Tofu, extra firm, 4 (16-ounce) blocks
- Tomatoes (6 large)

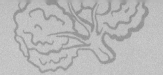

	MON — DAY 1	TUES — DAY 2	WEDS — DAY 3
breakfast	Sunflower-Oat Granola (page 76) + Almond Oat Milk (page 168) + fresh fruit *or* Endurance Smoothie (page 74) + 1 slice Bird Bread (page 164)	Sunflower-Oat Granola + Almond Oat Milk + fresh fruit *or* Endurance Smoothie + 1 slice Bird Bread	Sunflower-Oat Granola + Almond Oat Milk + fresh fruit *or* Endurance Smoothie + 1 slice Bird Bread
lunch	Moroccan Carrot Salad (page 94)	Leftover Saucy Slaw Bowl + Coconut-Crusted Tofu + Coconut Rice	Peach & Pepper Gazpacho (page 92) + 1 slice leftover Bird Bread
dinner	Saucy Slaw Bowl (page 112) + Coconut-Crusted Tofu (page 163) + Coconut Rice (page 155) or prepared brown rice	Peach & Sweet Potato Salad (page 113) (make enough for leftovers to have Thursday night)	Sloppy Joe Lentil-Stuffed Peppers (page 122) (make enough to eat again on Saturday)
snack	1 apple	Crispy Chickpeas (page 150)	Crispy Chickpeas

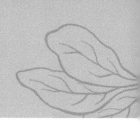

THURS DAY 4	FRI DAY 5	SAT DAY 6	SUN DAY 7
Sunflower-Oat Granola + Almond Oat Milk + fresh fruit *or* Endurance Smoothie + 1 slice Bird Bread	Sunflower-Oat Granola + Almond Oat Milk + fresh fruit *or* Endurance Smoothie + 1 slice Bird Bread	Sunrise Scramble (page 77)	Avocado Breakfast Boats (page 79)
Leftover Moroccan Carrot Salad	Leftover Peach & Pepper Gazpacho + 1 slice Bird Bread	Sloppy Joe Salad (cut up leftover Sloppy Joe Lentil-Stuffed Peppers and serve over greens)	Leftover Killer Tofu Kebabs over greens
Leftover Peach & Sweet Potato Salad	Date & Almond Kale Salad (page 123)	Killer Tofu Kebabs (page 120) + Coconut Rice	Olive & Herb Stuffed Tomatoes (page 114) (make enough to have for lunch tomorrow)
1 apple	Crispy Chickpeas	1 apple	1 apple

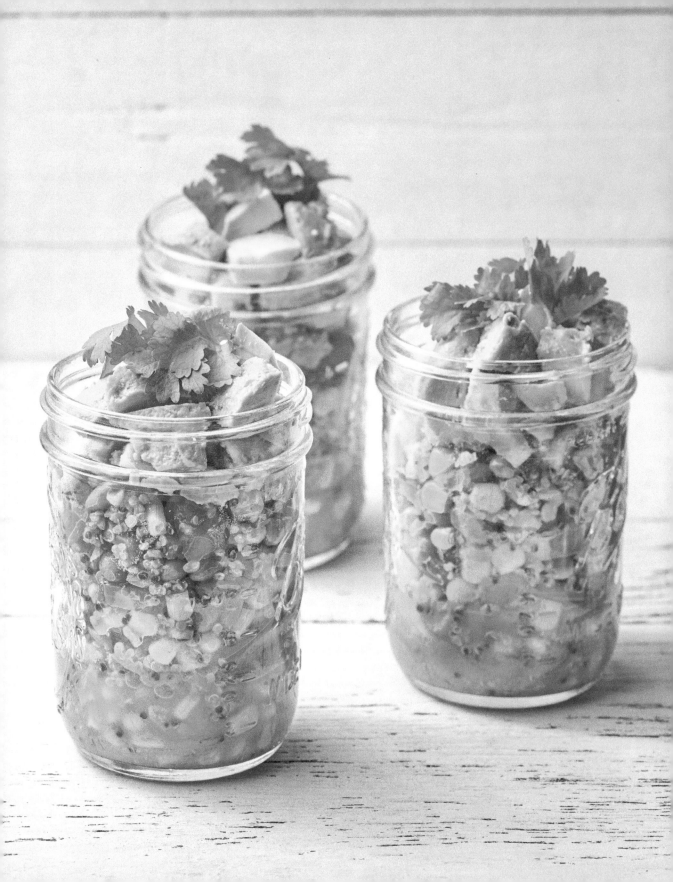

week two

Are you feeling so much better now than a week ago? Week 1 might have been a difficult adjustment, but you made it, so this is a great time to check in and take note of how you feel. Jot down any immediate benefits you have noticed, as these will fuel your motivation to continue. During week 2, you'll be introduced to more new flavors and preparations of old favorites. Again, make this work for you by swapping meals around and exchanging like ingredients (sweet potato for squash, or broccoli for cauliflower) when needed to make your life easier. If you had a favorite meal or snack from last week, repeat it this week, but remember that it will be fun for you to branch out and try all the recipes in this book.

OPPOSITE: BREAKFAST BURRITO JARS, PAGE 85

PREP AHEAD

Remember how much easier it was to eat well last week because you had some key items on hand, ready to go? Let's do that again this week.

For week 2, prepare the following items ahead of time:

- Super Seed & Nut Butter (page 169)
- Breakfast Burrito Jars (page 85)
- Peppery Pesto (page 176)
- Brown rice

- 2 baked sweet potatoes per person
- Stuffed Snacking Dates (page 148)

WEEK 2 SHOPPING LIST

Check your pantry, refrigerator, and freezer to see what you already have.

pantry

- Beans and legumes, canned: great northern, pinto, and yellow lentils
- Coconut aminos or tamari
- Coconut, unsweetened shredded
- Fruit, dried: blueberries and dates
- Grains: brown rice, oats, and quinoa
- Herbs and spices, dried: cardamom (ground), cayenne pepper (ground), chili powder, dukkah, Chinese five-spice powder, cinnamon (ground), cumin (ground), ginger (ground), red pepper flakes, and turmeric (ground)
- Nuts, raw: almonds, cashews, pine nuts, and walnuts
- Oils: coconut, extra-virgin olive, toasted sesame, and walnut

- Olives, Kalamata
- Seeds: chia, flax, hemp, sesame, and sunflower
- Supplements (optional): cacao powder, collagen powder, nutritional yeast, and/or protein powder
- Sweeteners: honey and maple syrup
- Tahini
- Tomatoes, canned
- Tomatoes, sun-dried
- Vinegar: apple cider, balsamic, and white balsamic

refrigerator/freezer

- Apples (3)
- Arugula (2 containers)
- Avocado (2)
- Bananas (5)
- Basil (1 bunch)
- Broccoli (2)
- Carrots (1 pound)
- Cilantro (1 bunch)
- Corn, kernels, frozen or fresh (8 ounce)
- Cucumber
- Edamame, frozen (1 package)
- Garlic (1 head)
- Ginger (1 knob)
- Greens, mixed (1 large container)
- Kale, lacinato (2 bunches)
- Lemons (2)
- Lettuce, iceberg (2)
- Lettuce, romaine (2)
- Limes (3)
- Mint (2 bunches)
- Nut milk of choice (1 container)
- Onion, yellow (1)
- Onions, red (3)
- Oranges, mandarin (2)
- Parsley (2 bunches)
- Pepper, red chile (1)
- Peppers, jalapeño (2)
- Peppers, red bell (4)
- Pineapple, chunks (1 bag)
- Potatoes, sweet (2)
- Scallions (1 bunch)
- Shallot (1)
- Squash, summer (4 large)
- Tempeh (1 [8-ounce] package)
- Tofu, extra firm (2 [16-ounce] packages)
- Tomatoes (8 large)
- Zucchini (4 large)

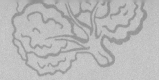

	MON DAY 8	TUES DAY 9	WEDS DAY 10
breakfast	Breakfast Burrito Jar (page 85) *or* Super Seed & Nut Butter Smoothie (page 73)	Breakfast Burrito Jar *or* Super Seed & Nut Butter Smoothie	Breakfast Burrito Jar *or* Super Seed & Nut Butter Smoothie
lunch	Chop up last night's leftover Olive & Herb Stuffed Tomatoes and serve over greens	Cool & Crunchy Chop (page 103)	Leftover Killer Tofu Kebabs + mixed greens + quinoa or rice
dinner	Grilled Zucchini Salad (page 118)	Killer Tofu Kebabs (page 120) (make enough for Wednesday's lunch)	Date & Almond Kale Salad (page 123)
snack	Stuffed Snacking Dates (page 148)	1 banana	Stuffed Snacking Dates

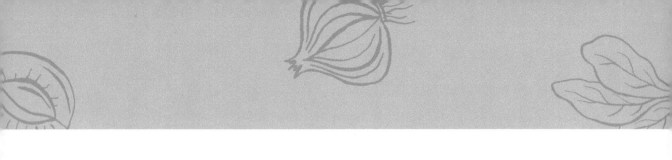

THURS DAY 11	FRI DAY 12	SAT DAY 13	SUN DAY 14
Breakfast Burrito Jar *or* Super Seed & Nut Butter Smoothie	Breakfast Burrito Jar *or* Super Seed & Nut Butter Smoothie	Dirty Chai Overnight Oats (page 78)	Tempeh Sausage Patties (page 87)
Leftover Cool & Crunchy Chop	Leftover Fitness Fried Rice + Fruit	Warm Bean & Tomato Toss (page 96)	Leftover Cool & Crunchy Chop
Fitness Fried Rice (page 162)	Pesto Non-Pasta (page 124)	Detox Bowls (page 121)	Lentil & Vegetable Curry (page 130) (make enough for Monday's lunch)
1 banana	Stuffed Snacking Dates	Stuffed Snacking Dates	1 banana

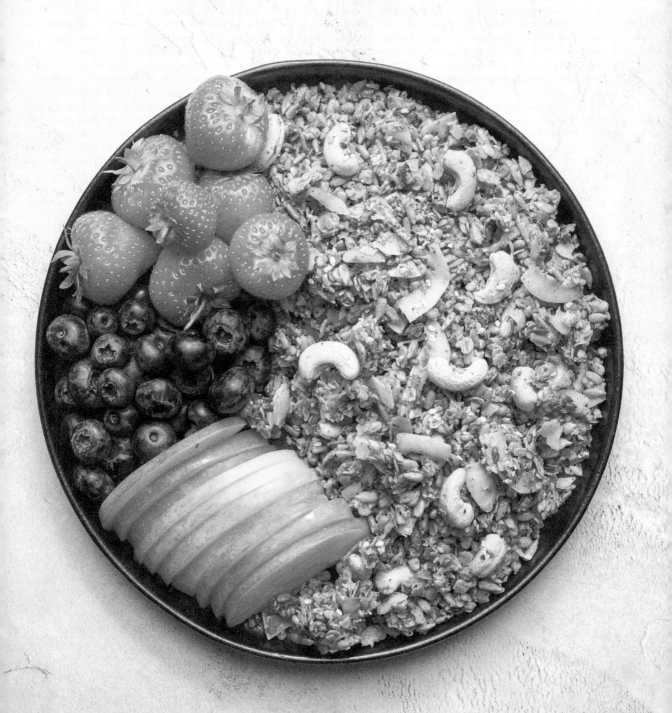

CHAPTER FIVE

week three

Another week down and you're going strong. Taking this journey is an incredible step in self-care and health promotion. By now you've likely settled into your new routine and are feeling comfortable and confident eating whole foods daily. Check in with yourself again this week. Note your hunger levels, energy, skin condition, digestion, sleep, and any other positive quality of life changes. Week 3 will repeat a few items from the previous two weeks and introduce new ingredients, combinations, and recipes. If you have leftovers, try to mix and match different sides, snacks, and meals to create your own unique favorites. Getting through this week puts you over the halfway hump—you can do it!

OPPOSITE: SUNFLOWER-OAT GRANOLA, PAGE 76

PREP AHEAD

Before getting started this week, take stock of what you have on hand. Any leftover meals or ingredients can be included this week to reduce the shopping and work-load. For example, if you have assorted vegetables, dice them and toss into a broth with beans for a quick soup, or if there are extra Tempeh Sausage Patties (page 87), crumble them over greens for a lunch salad.

For week 3 prepare the following items ahead of time:

- Bird Bread (page 164)
- Dirty Chai Overnight Oats (page 78)
- 24-Carrot Hummus (page 157)
- Energizing Trail Mix (page 159)

WEEK 3 SHOPPING LIST

Check your pantry, refrigerator, and freezer to see what you already have.

pantry

- Banana chips
- Beans and legumes, canned: black and chickpeas
- Coconut, unsweetened shredded
- Coconut aminos or tamari
- Coffee
- Fruit, dried: apricots, goji berries, and golden raisins
- Grains: brown rice, oats, and quinoa
- Herbs and spices, dried: Balti, cardamom (ground), caraway seeds, cayenne pepper (ground), cinnamon (ground), cumin (ground), curry powder, dukkah, ginger (ground), poppy seeds, red pepper flakes, and turmeric (ground)
- Nuts, raw: almonds, cashews, and peanuts
- Oils: avocado, coconut, extra-virgin olive, toasted sesame, and walnut
- Olives
- Psyllium powder

- Seeds: chia, flax (seed and meal), hemp, pumpkin, sesame, and sunflower
- Supplements (optional): collagen powder, nutritional yeast, and/or protein powder
- Spirulina
- Sweeteners: honey and maple syrup
- Tahini
- Vinegars: apple cider, balsamic, and white balsamic

refrigerator/freezer

- Apples (3)
- Avocado (2)
- Bananas (4)
- Basil (1 bunch)
- Carrots (1 pound)
- Chives (1 bunch)
- Cilantro (3 bunches)
- Cucumber, English (1)
- Garlic (1 head)
- Ginger (1 knob)
- Greens, mixed (1 large container)
- Kale (1 bunch)
- Lemons (3)
- Limes (6)
- Mint (1 bunch)
- Nut milk of choice (1 container)
- Onions, red (3)
- Onion, yellow (1)
- Orange (1)
- Parsley (6 bunches)
- Pepper, jalapeño (3)
- Peppers, orange bell (1)
- Peppers, red bell (2)
- Pineapple, chunks, frozen (1 bag)
- Scallions (1 bunch)
- Shallot (1)
- Spinach (2 cups)
- Squash, summer (4 large)
- Sweet potato (1)
- Tofu, extra firm (3 [16-ounce] blocks)
- Tomatoes, cherry (1 pint)
- Zucchini (4 large)

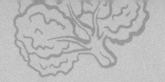

	MON DAY 15	**TUES** DAY 16	**WEDS** DAY 17
breakfast	Dirty Chai Overnight Oats (page 78) *or* Kale & Banana Smoothie (page 72)	Dirty Chai Overnight Oats *or* Kale & Banana Smoothie	Dirty Chai Overnight Oats *or* Kale & Banana Smoothie
lunch	Leftover Lentil & Vegetable Curry over rice or greens	Crunchy Tahini Toast (page 97)	Leftover Grilled Zucchini Salad with Crispy Chickpeas (page 150)
dinner	Grilled Zucchini Salad (page 118) (make enough for lunch later in the week)	Falafel Bowls (page 128) (make enough for Friday lunch)	Detox Bowls (page 121)
snack	Energizing Trail Mix (page 159)	Energizing Trail Mix	Energizing Trail Mix

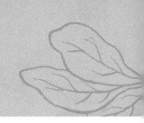

THURS DAY 18	FRI DAY 19	SAT DAY 20	SUN DAY 21
Dirty Chai Overnight Oats *or* Kale & Banana Smoothie	Dirty Chai Overnight Oats *or* Kale & Banana Smoothie	Sunrise Scramble (page 77) + Golden Leo Latte (page 152)	Leftover Sunrise Scramble + nut milk + fresh fruit
Chickpea Salad Toast (page 95) or Crunchy Tahini Toast (page 97)	Leftover Falafel Bowls over Massaged Kale (page 151)	Leftover Chickpea Salad Toast	Leftover Killer Tofu Kebabs, chopped and stir-fried with sweet potato
Mixed Grill Bowls (page 116)	Killer Tofu Kebabs (page 120) (make enough for Sunday lunch) + Coconut Rice (page 155)	Use up your leftovers. Toss veggies and sweet potatoes with Massaged Kale	Leftover Detox Bowls
Energizing Trail Mix	1 apple	Energizing Trail Mix	Energizing Trail Mix

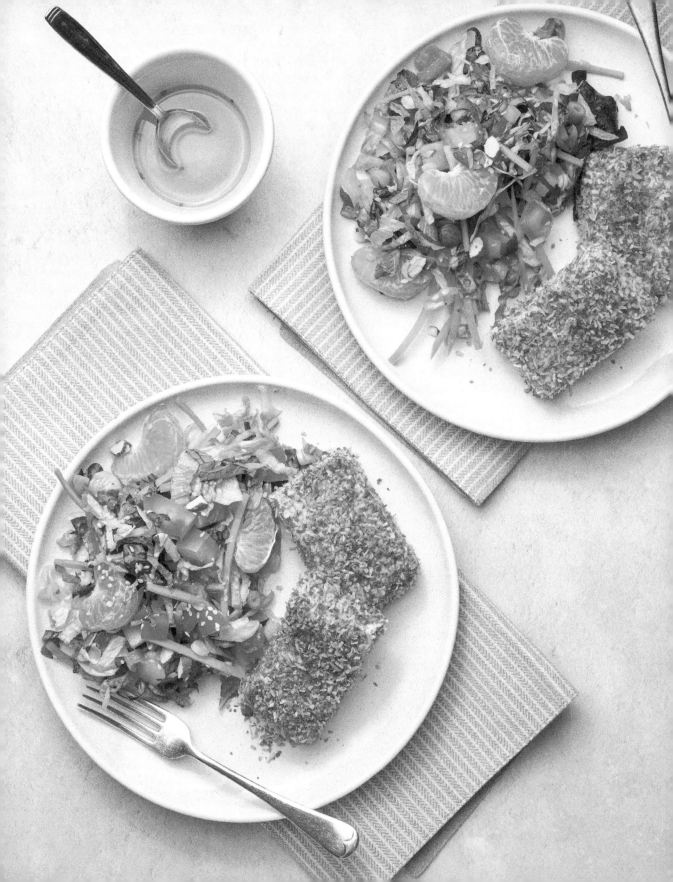

week four

Just pause for a moment and congratulate yourself. By getting to week 4 of the plan, you've really put in serious effort and energy to improve your well-being. This is a big deal, and it should be celebrated. Before starting this week, jot down a few highlights you've experienced thus far, such as favorite meals, moments (having a coworker compliment your newfound glow or no longer craving a sugar snack), etc. These moments are big milestones and should be remembered for future encouragement to stick with a plant-forward, whole food eating plan. For this final full week, I'm throwing in some of my favorite go-to recipes so you can really experience how delicious whole foods are. After this it's going to be really hard for you to stop eating this way.

OPPOSITE: COOL & CRUNCHY CHOP, PAGE 103
AND COCONUT-CRUSTED TOFU, PAGE 163

PREP AHEAD

By now, you're getting the hang of making your own meals so there is less to prep ahead of time.

For week 4, prepare the following items ahead of time:

- Sunflower-Oat Granola (page 76)
- Spicy "Cheesy" Cashew Sauce (page 178)

- Creamy Balsamic Dressing (page 174)
- Cooked grain of choice
- Almond Oat Milk (page 168)

WEEK 4 SHOPPING LIST

Check your pantry, refrigerator, and freezer to see what you already have.

pantry

- Beans and legumes, canned: black, chickpeas, great northern, and white
- Coconut aminos or tamari
- Coconut milk, canned
- Coconut, unsweetened shredded
- Fruit, dried: blueberries and dates
- Ghee
- Grains: brown rice, oats, and quinoa
- Herbs and spices, dried: cardamom (ground), cayenne pepper (ground), Chinese five-spice powder, chipotle pepper flakes, cinnamon (ground), cumin (ground), curry powder, ginger (ground), oregano, poppy seeds, red pepper flakes, sage, and turmeric (ground)

- Maple syrup
- Nut butter
- Nuts, raw: almonds, cashews, pine nuts, walnuts
- Oils: avocado, coconut, extra-virgin olive, toasted sesame, and walnut
- Olives, Kalamata
- Raisins
- Salsa, corn and bean
- Seeds: chia, flax (seeds and meal), hemp, pumpkin seeds, sesame, sunflower
- Supplements (optional): collagen powder, nutritional yeast, and/or protein powder
- Sweeteners: honey and maple syrup
- Tahini

- Tomatoes, canned
- Vanilla extract

- Vinegars: apple cider, red and white balsamic, rice

refrigerator/freezer

- Apples (6)
- Arugula (1 container)
- Avocado (5)
- Bananas (2)
- Basil (1 bunch)
- Broccoli (2)
- Carrots (1 pound)
- Chives (1 bunch)
- Cilantro (1 bunch)
- Corn tortillas (8)
- Corn, kernels, frozen (8 ounces)
- Cucumber (2)
- Dill (1 bunch)
- Edamame, frozen (1 package)
- Eggs, large (1 dozen)
- Garlic (1 head)
- Ginger (1 knob)
- Jicama (1)
- Kale, lacinato (2 bunches)
- Lemons (2)
- Lettuce, iceberg (1)
- Lettuce, romaine (1 large head)
- Lime (1)
- Mint (2 bunches)
- Nut milk of choice (1 container)
- Onion, sweet (1)
- Onions, red (5)
- Oranges, mandarin (2)
- Parsley (1 bunch)
- Peas, English (1 cup)
- Peppers, red bell (6)
- Peppers, yellow bell (1)
- Potatoes, sweet (4)
- Potatoes, Yukon Gold (2)
- Rosemary (1 bunch)
- Scallions (1 bunch)
- Shallots (2)
- Tempeh (1 [8-ounce] package)
- Tofu, extra firm (4 [16-ounce] blocks)
- Tomatoes (7 large)
- Zucchini (2 large)

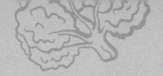

	MON DAY 22	TUES DAY 23	WEDS DAY 24
breakfast	Sunflower-Oat Granola (page 76) + Almond Oat Milk (page 168) + fresh fruit *or* Savory Sweet Potato Toast (page 80)	Sunflower-Oat Granola + Almond Oat Milk + fresh fruit *or* Leftover Savory Sweet Potato Toast	Sunflower-Oat Granola + Almond Oat Milk + fresh fruit *or* Leftover Savory Sweet Potato Toast
lunch	Green Quinoa Salad (page 90)	Taco Salad (page 105)	Warm Bean & Tomato Toss (page 96)
dinner	Date & Almond Kale Salad (page 123)	Grilled Zucchini Salad (page 118) + brown rice	"Cheesy" Broccoli & Rice (page 131)
snack	1 apple	Golden Leo Latte (page 152)	1 apple

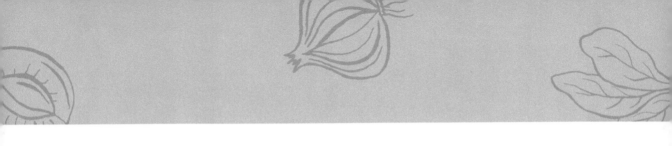

THURS DAY 25	FRI DAY 26	SAT DAY 27	SUN DAY 28
Sunflower-Oat Granola + Almond Oat Milk + fresh fruit *or* Leftover Savory Sweet Potato Toast	Sunflower-Oat Granola + Almond Oat Milk + fresh fruit *or* Leftover Savory Sweet Potato Toast	Avocado Breakfast Boats (page 79)	Tempeh Sausage Patties (page 87) (make enough to carry you into next week) + fresh fruit
Leftover Green Quinoa Salad	"Cheesy" Quesadillas (page 109)	Leftover Sloppy Joe Lentil-Stuffed Peppers (cut them up and serve over greens or with sweet potatoes)	Cool & Crunchy Chop (page 103) + Coconut-Crusted Tofu
Fitness Fried Rice (page 162) + Coconut-Crusted Tofu (page 163) (make enough to eat again Sunday evening)	Sloppy Joe Lentil-Stuffed Peppers (page 122) (make enough to eat again Saturday lunch	Date & Almond Kale Salad	Fitness Fried Rice + Leftover Coconut-Crusted Tofu
Golden Leo Latte	1 apple	Golden Leo Latte	1 apple

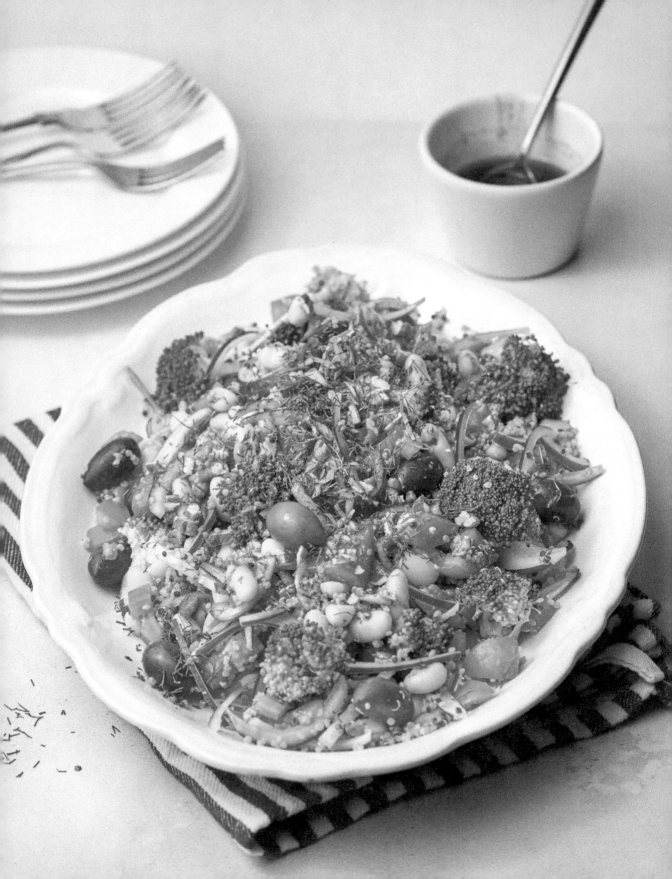

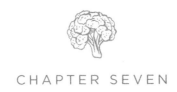

week five

Just two days left! Take a deep breath and smile. Let it sink in that you're about to finish a 30-day commitment. Reflect on all the work that went into this and how much you've enjoyed the process. Again, take note of those quality of life changes. Do you weigh less than in week 1? Smile more? Sleep deeper? While you might be doing this for serious disease prevention, those results are a bit harder to notice, and at this time it helps to pay attention to what you can measure as results. Try getting your numbers (blood pressure, cholesterol, and body fat) from your physician to see what improvements you've made from implementing this plan.

OPPOSITE: WARM BEAN & TOMATO TOSS, PAGE 96

PREP AHEAD

For these final two days, try a new recipe that hasn't yet really pushed your bound-aries in terms of new tastes. Preparing extra meals and batches of granola, grains, and dressings will help carry your new habits beyond these final couple days.

For week 5, prepare the following items ahead of time:

- Avocado Breakfast Boats (page 79)
- Golden Tahini Dressing (page 172)
- Brown rice

- Almond Oat Milk (page 168)
- Energizing Trail Mix (page 159)

WEEK 5 SHOPPING LIST

Check your pantry, refrigerator, and freezer to see what you already have.

pantry

- Beans and legumes, canned: great northern
- Coconut, unsweetened shredded
- Fruit, dried: apricots, banana chips, dates, goji berries
- Grains: brown rice, oats, quinoa
- Herbs and spices, dried: Balti seasoning or garam marsala, cardamom (ground), cayenne pepper (ground), cumin (ground), curry powder, dukkah, ginger (ground), paprika, poppy seeds, red pepper flakes, and turmeric (ground)
- Miso paste, white
- Nuts, raw: almonds, cashews, peanuts, and walnuts

- Oils: coconut, extra-virgin olive, and toasted sesame
- Olives, Kalamata
- Seeds: chia, flax, hemp, pumpkin, sesame, and sunflower
- Supplements (optional): collagen powder, nutritional yeast, and/or protein powder
- Sweeteners: honey and maple syrup
- Tahini
- Coconut aminos or tamari
- Vanilla extract
- Vinegars: apple cider, red and white balsamic

refrigerator/freezer

- Apples (3)
- Arugula (1)
- Avocados (4)
- Bananas (4)
- Broccoli (1)
- Garlic (1 head)
- Mushrooms (16 ounces)
- Nut milk of choice (1 container)
- Onion, red (1)
- Parsley (1 bunch)
- Pepper, jalapeño (1)
- Potato, sweet (1)
- Spinach (1 container)
- Tofu, extra firm (2 [16-ounce] blocks)
- Tomatoes (3 large)

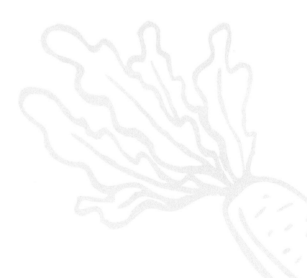

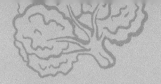

	MON DAY 29	TUES DAY 30
breakfast	Avocado Breakfast Boats (page 79) + Almond Oat Milk (page 168)+ fresh fruit	Avocado Breakfast Boats + Almond Oat Milk + fresh fruit
lunch	Leftover Tempeh Sausage Patties + greens with Golden Tahini Dressing (page 172)	Warm Bean & Tomato Toss (page 96)
dinner	Detox Bowl (page 121)	Miso-Mushroom Stir-Fry (page 117)
snack	Energizing Trail Mix (page 159)	1 apple

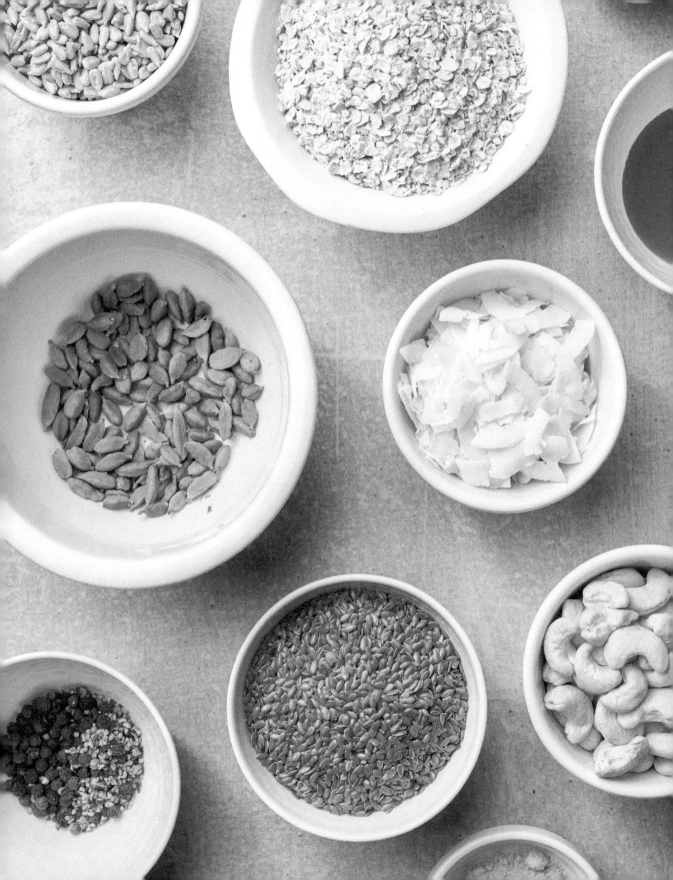

AFTER 30 DAYS

Right now, you're likely feeling great about your accomplishment and what this practice did for your well-being. Let the feeling soak in because you earned it! You just completed 30 days of plant-forward, whole food eating, which is no small feat. You learned to shop for ingredients and cook meals that will increase your health, well-being, and quality of life. You implemented new healthy habits and ditched foods that were holding you back from reaching your goals, and you did it for a full 30 days. Doesn't that feel good?

reintroducing foods

Now that you've finished the 30 days, it is time to look beyond and think about what comes next. If you're ready to reintroduce foods that weren't consumed on this plan, start slowly. Add back small amounts of dairy, meat, poultry, fish, eggs, and minimally processed foods (chickpea pasta, sprouted bread, etc.). The key is to limit these items and treat them as condiments to your whole, nourishing plant foods. When you add back a food, pay close attention to how your body feels. If you reintroduce a food you haven't eaten in weeks, and it causes headaches, fogginess, gastric distress, skin rashes, cravings, or moodiness, you might have a food sensitivity and should consider limiting or avoiding that food permanently.

For long-term success, it is important to bend the rules a little; eat out with friends, grab a snack on the go, treat yourself, and so on. The more your regular diet resembles this meal plan most of the time, the less occasionally treating yourself can harm your overall health.

Remember those notes you were encouraged to take while following the meal plan? Consult them as you move on. Compare the feelings you had on versus off the meal plan. Focusing on how you felt on the 30-day whole foods diet meal plan and how you feel returning to more normal eating should motivate you to continue your new healthy habits.

continuing

The 30th day is the "end" of this meal plan, but it doesn't have to be the end of your whole food-based eating. You can add another round of 30 days to really make these habits stick and increase the benefits you see and feel. There are plenty of recipes in this book to choose from to create your own meal plan, or just repeat the meal plan provided. A good way of moving forward is to plan 30 days of a loosened-up version to transition out of the stricter plan while still continuing healthy eating. Simply use the recipes provided in the book, adding in a few of your favorite high-quality animal products or lightly processed ingredients (eggs, feta, and salmon, for example). If you need to step away from the plan completely, remember the benefits you gained from your first 30 days, and if at any point you feel your health and good habits starting to slip, just restart the 30 days to get back on track.

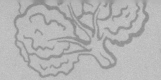

	monday	tuesday	wednesday
breakfast			
lunch			
dinner			
Snack			

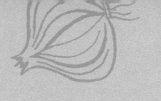
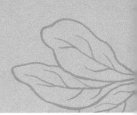

thursday	friday	saturday	sunday

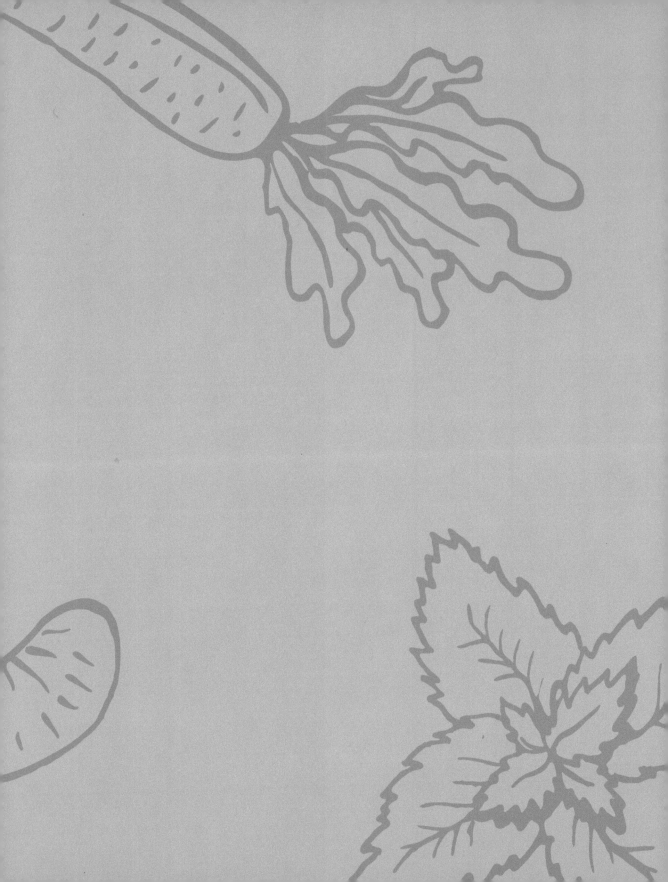

recipes

Like in any meal plan, there may be things you cannot eat due to ingredient seasonality, time available, food allergy, intolerance, or personal preference. That is why this section contains ample whole food recipes that are simple to prepare and will make a big impact on your health. While many of the recipes are included in the meal plan, there are plenty more that are not, so have fun looking through them. Allow yourself to make recipe swaps based on what works best for you throughout the 30-day commitment. After the 30 days, use this section as you would use any recipe book to experiment with new flavors, simple meals, and nutrient-rich, whole food options.

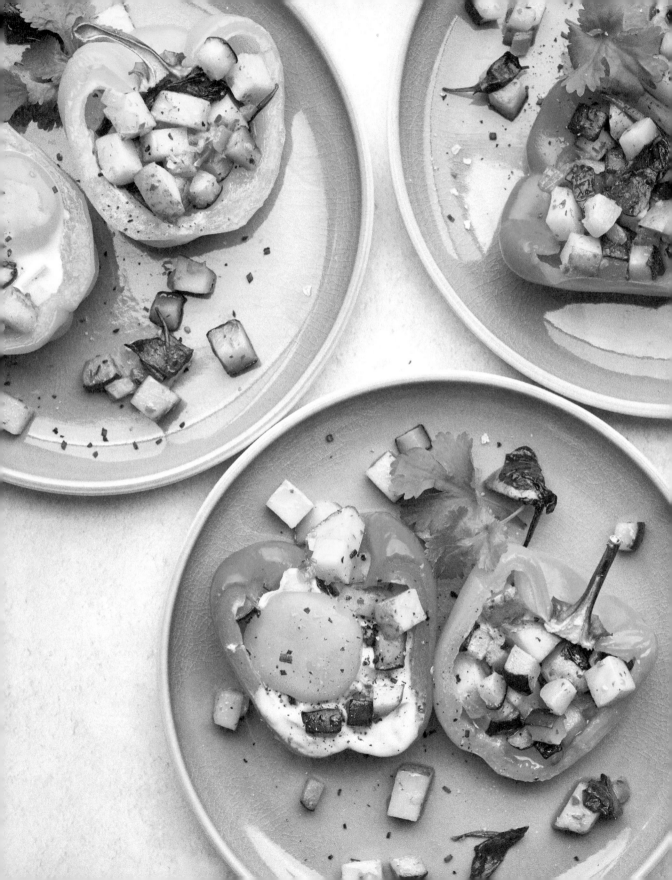

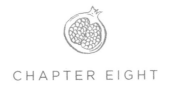

CHAPTER EIGHT

breakfast

OPPOSITE: BREAKFAST STUFFED PEPPERS, PAGE 86

kale & banana smoothie

DAIRY-FREE, FREEZER-FRIENDLY, GLUTEN-FREE,
GRAIN-FREE, QUICK, VEGAN

serves: 4 | serving size: 1½ cups
prep time: 5 minutes | cook time: n/a

Adding greens to your morning smoothie is a great way to start the day with a vibrant boost. Frozen kale is great here. This cooling, satisfying blend helps give you a little pep.

---

4 dates, pitted

4 cups almond milk (or any dairy-free milk)

2 cups kale

4 ripe bananas

1 avocado, peeled and pitted

Pinch salt

Pinch spirulina (optional)

Ice or water (optional)

1. In a blender, pulse the dates until broken up.

2. Add the milk, kale, bananas, avocado, salt, and spirulina (if using), and blend until smooth.

3. Add ice or water to increase the volume if desired, blend again, pour into glasses, and serve.

super seed & nut butter smoothie

DAIRY-FREE, FREEZER-FRIENDLY, GLUTEN-FREE,
GRAIN-FREE, QUICK, VEGAN

serves: 4 | serving size: 2 cups
prep time: 5 minutes | cook time: n/a

I love using smoothies as a vessel to get all my nutrients in one drink. They get me nourished, energized, and out the door ASAP.

6 cups almond milk (or any dairy-free milk)

2 cups frozen cauliflower florets

2 cups cubed cooked sweet potato

¼ cup Super Seed & Nut Butter (page 169)

1 teaspoon vanilla extract

Ice or water (optional)

1. In a blender, combine the milk, cauliflower, sweet potato, Super Seed & Nut Butter, and vanilla.

2. Blend until smooth.

3. Add ice or water to increase the volume if desired, blend again, pour into glasses, and serve.

endurance smoothie

DAIRY-FREE, FREEZER-FRIENDLY, GLUTEN-FREE, GRAIN-FREE,
NUT-FREE, QUICK, VEGETARIAN

serves: 4 | serving size: 1½ cups
prep time: 5 minutes | cook time: n/a

In my healthy, well-nourished world, a winning smoothie is one that refreshes, hydrates, and energizes with lasting nutrients. This one is like a coconut-orange creamsicle with B vitamins from the bee pollen to energize and good fats to keep you satisfied.

---

2 avocados, peeled and pitted

2 bananas

2 cups fresh orange juice

2 cups coconut milk

2 cups coconut water

2 tablespoons coconut oil

1 tablespoon bee pollen

1 tablespoon hemp seeds

Ice (optional)

1. In a blender, combine the avocados, bananas, orange juice, coconut milk, coconut water, coconut oil, bee pollen, and hemp seeds, and blend until smooth.

2. Add ice to the blender if desired, blend again, pour into glasses, and serve.

kiwi-berry smoothie

DAIRY-FREE, FREEZER-FRIENDLY, GLUTEN-FREE, GRAIN-FREE,
NUT-FREE, QUICK, VEGETARIAN

serves: 4 | serving size: 1½ cups
prep time: 5 minutes | cook time: n/a

Did you know the skin of a kiwi is edible? Give yourself some extra fiber (and reduce prep time) by leaving the peel on. Make smoothies a lot faster by freezing the chopped ingredients in freezer-safe bags. This way, you can just take out a portion pack, add liquid, and blend.

4 cups water
4 kiwis, chopped
1 cup raspberries
1 avocado, peeled and pitted
1 cup frozen young coconut meat
¼ cup honey

In a blender, combine the water, kiwis, raspberries, avocado, coconut, and honey. Blend until smooth, pour into glasses, and serve.

sunflower-oat granola

DAIRY-FREE, GLUTEN-FREE, QUICK, VEGAN

serves: 12 | serving size: ½ cup
prep time: 5 minutes
cook time: 10 minutes, plus 15 minutes to cool

I could (and do) snack on this granola by the handful. There is always a jar in my pantry, and whenever it gets low, I quickly make another batch. Sometimes I'll add dried fruit or different nuts, like pecans instead of cashews, depending on what I have on hand.

---

2 cups old-fashioned oats

1 cup unsweetened coconut

¼ cup coconut oil

¼ cup flaxseed

2 cups raw sunflower seeds

1 cup raw cashews

2 tablespoons untoasted sesame seeds

1 teaspoon salt

1 teaspoon ground ginger

½ teaspoon ground cardamom

½ cup maple syrup

¼ cup supplements, such as maca, baobab, lucuma, or protein (optional)

1. In a large skillet over medium heat, toast the oats, stirring, until golden, about 5 minutes.

2. Add the coconut and stir frequently until golden and fragrant. This happens quickly, so stay by the stove, stirring often.

3. Immediately reduce the heat to low and add the coconut oil, flaxseed, sunflower seeds, cashews, sesame seeds, salt, ginger, and cardamom.

4. Stir well to combine.

5. Pour in the maple syrup, and stir to coat.

6. Cook for about 1 minute, then remove from the heat and stir in the supplements, if using.

7. Let sit for about 15 minutes to firm up and cool completely before serving or storing.

8. Store in an airtight container in your pantry for up to 2 weeks.

sunrise scramble

DAIRY-FREE, GLUTEN-FREE, GRAIN-FREE, NUT-FREE, QUICK, VEGAN

serves: 4 | serving size: ¼ of recipe
prep time: 10 minutes | cook time: 15 minutes

On days when you have a little extra time and need a filling meal, this dish is a must. If a curry-like flavor isn't your thing, just swap those spices for a milder herby blend. Balti seasoning is a spicy blend of herbs and spices from northern Pakistan. If you can't find it, use harissa, chermoula, or dukkah.

1 tablespoon coconut oil

1 cup finely chopped red onion

1 sweet potato, shredded (or use leftover cooked sweet potato)

1 (16-ounce) firm or extra-firm block tofu, drained and patted dry

2 garlic cloves, minced

2 teaspoons ground turmeric

2 teaspoons Balti seasoning

1 teaspoon salt

½ teaspoon freshly ground black pepper

2 cups spinach

¼ cup nutritional yeast

Chopped avocado or tomatoes (optional)

1. In a large skillet over medium heat, heat the coconut oil.

2. Add the onion and sweet potato and cook for 3 to 4 minutes, until the onion softens slightly.

3. Crumble the tofu into the skillet, using your fingers.

4. Add the garlic, turmeric, Balti seasoning, salt, and pepper and cook, stirring occasionally, for about 10 minutes.

5. Stir in the spinach, cooking until wilted.

6. Remove from the heat, sprinkle with the nutritional yeast, and serve.

7. Add avocado or chopped tomatoes, if using.

dirty chai overnight oats

DAIRY-FREE, GLUTEN-FREE, VEGETARIAN

serves: 4 | serving size: 1½ cups
prep time: 5 minutes plus overnight to set
cook time: n/a

For those days when you need a morning energy burst but can't decide between coffee or tea, this blend provides it all: a hearty jar of oats with a spiced jolt of caffeine. It's my favorite breakfast on busy days.

---

2 cups almond milk (or any dairy-free milk)

2 cups cold brew coffee

¼ cup honey

¼ cup tahini

½ teaspoon ground cinnamon

½ teaspoon ground ginger

½ teaspoon ground cardamom

¼ teaspoon salt

2 cups old-fashioned oats

2 bananas, sliced

Fresh fruit, chopped nuts, unsweetened shredded coconut, or cacao nibs, for topping (optional)

1. In a blender, combine the milk, coffee, honey, tahini, cinnamon, ginger, cardamom, and salt.

2. In a large bowl, stir the spiced coffee blend together with the oats and sliced bananas.

3. Scoop into 4 jars and cover.

4. Place in the refrigerator overnight.

5. In the morning, add your topping (if using), grab a jar, and go.

avocado breakfast boats

DAIRY-FREE, GLUTEN-FREE, GRAIN-FREE, QUICK, VEGAN

serves: 4 | serving size: ½ avocado
prep time: 10 minutes | cook time: n/a

Call it a strange combo, but I love avocado and nut butter sandwiches. Yum! It reminds me of going to school and packing lunch, but in a grown-up way. This recipe lets you ditch the bread and still retain the flavor.

2 bananas, chopped

¼ cup Super Seed & Nut Butter (page 169)

2 avocados, halved and pitted

½ tablespoon hemp seeds

½ tablespoon flaxseed

1. In a medium bowl, mix the banana chunks together with the Super Seed & Nut Butter.

2. Place a scoop of the banana mixture into each avocado half.

3. Top each with a sprinkle of hemp and flaxseed and serve.

savory sweet potato toast

DAIRY-FREE, GLUTEN-FREE, GRAIN-FREE, MAKE AHEAD,
NUT-FREE, VEGETARIAN

serves: 4 | serving size: 2 slices
prep time: 10 minutes | cook time: 25 minutes

Forget bread. Sweet potatoes are a great source of complex carbohydrates and nutrients. Once you master the technique, get creative with your toppings.

2 sweet potatoes, cut lengthwise into
   ¼-inch-thick slices

1 avocado

4 hard-boiled eggs (optional)

1 cup corn and bean salsa

Pinch salt (optional)

Pinch chipotle pepper flakes (optional)

1. Preheat the oven to 350°F.

2. Set a wire baking rack over a baking sheet. Lay each sweet potato slice on the wire rack.

3. Bake for 20 to 25 minutes, until the potato slices start to soften.

4. Remove from the oven. (Steps 1 through 4 can be completed ahead of time. Store the baked slices in the refrigerator to make morning sweet potato toast super quick.).

5. Toast each slice in a toaster.

6. In a medium bowl, mash the avocado together with the eggs (if using).

7. Top each sweet potato slice with a scoop of the salsa and avocado.

8. Sprinkle with salt and chipotle pepper flakes to taste (if using) and serve.

super sweet potato toast

DAIRY-FREE, GLUTEN-FREE, GRAIN-FREE, MAKE AHEAD, NUT-FREE, VEGAN

serves: 4 | serving size: 2 slices
prep time: 10 minutes | cook time: 30 minutes

Plant-based whole food doesn't have to be boring or lack sweetness. This toast is like a healthy dessert for breakfast.

---

2 sweet potatoes, cut lengthwise into ¼-inch-thick slices
½ tablespoon coconut oil
1 apple, diced
2 tablespoons maple syrup
Pinch ground cinnamon
Pinch salt
1 tablespoon chia seeds

1. Preheat the oven to 350°F.

2. Set a wire baking rack over a baking sheet. Lay each sweet potato slice on the wire rack.

3. Bake for 20 to 25 minutes, until the potato slices start to soften.

4. Remove from the oven. (Steps 1 through 4 can be completed ahead of time. Store the baked slices in the refrigerator to make morning sweet potato toast super quick.)

5. Toast each slice in a toaster.

6. Meanwhile, in a small skillet over medium heat, combine the coconut oil, apple, maple syrup, and cinnamon.

7. Sauté, stirring often until the apple is softened, about 5 minutes, then add the salt.

8. Top each sweet potato slice with the apple mixture, sprinkle with the chia seeds, and serve.

superfood smoothie bowls

DAIRY-FREE, GLUTEN-FREE, MAKE AHEAD, QUICK, VEGAN

serves: 4 | serving size: 2 cups
prep time: 10 minutes | cook time: n/a

This dish is a great reminder that green doesn't have to mean a salad. If I have a very busy day ahead, this is a go-to morning meal for me. It keeps me going strong for hours. I also love how customizable smoothie bowls are just by using different toppings. I can make this superfood base in advance and top with something new each morning.

2 zucchini

2 kiwis, peeled

2 bananas

1 avocado, peeled and pitted

8 pitted dates

2 cups coconut water

2 cups almond milk (or any dairy-free milk)

½ cup unsweetened shredded coconut

2 tablespoons cacao powder

1 tablespoon spirulina (optional but highly recommended)

1 teaspoon vanilla extract

½ teaspoon salt

Sunflower-Oat Granola (page 76), for topping

1. Roughly chop the zucchini, kiwis, bananas, avocado, and dates. (You can place all solid ingredients in a freezer-safe bag and freeze until ready to blend.)

2. In a blender, combine the chopped zucchini, kiwis, bananas, avocado, and dates with the coconut water, milk, shredded coconut, cacao powder, spirulina, vanilla, and salt, and blend until smooth.

3. Pour into bowls, top each bowl with a handful of granola, and serve.

power porridge

DAIRY-FREE, GLUTEN-FREE, MAKE AHEAD, QUICK, VEGETARIAN

serves: 4 | serving size: 1 cup
prep time: 10 minutes | cook time: 15 minutes

Wake up to the earthy taste of energizing matcha in a powerful grain bowl. This porridge can be made ahead and consumed warm or cold with a variety of toppings to keep things interesting and exciting (and use up whatever you have on hand).

2 cups coconut milk (or any dairy-free milk)

2 cups water

¼ cup honey

1 tablespoon coconut oil

2 teaspoons matcha powder

2 cups quinoa

Fresh fruit, nuts, hemp seeds, and/or shredded coconut, for topping

1. In a large saucepan over medium heat, combine the milk, water, honey, coconut oil, and matcha.

2. Whisk until the matcha and honey are incorporated into the milk and the coconut oil is melted.

3. Bring to simmer and reduce heat to low. Do not boil.

4. Add the quinoa to the pot and simmer until tender, about 15 minutes.

5. Portion into bowls, add desired toppings, and serve.

sunshine pudding

DAIRY-FREE, GLUTEN-FREE, MAKE AHEAD, VEGETARIAN

serves: 4 | serving size: 1 cup
prep time: 10 minutes, plus at least 2 hours to set
cook time: n/a

Mornings can be a chaotic rush to get out the door. I love breakfast recipes that can be mostly prepared the night before to make sure I have something healthy ready to grab and go. These bright, anti-inflammatory "pudding" cups are great for these situations.

---

2 cups coconut milk (or any dairy-free milk)
6 tablespoons chia seeds
2 teaspoons vanilla extract
1 cup frozen mango chunks
1 cup frozen pineapple chunks
1 teaspoon ground turmeric
½ teaspoon ground ginger
¼ cup honey
Sunflower-Oat Granola (page 76), bee pollen, chopped nuts, banana, and/or unsweetened shredded coconut, for topping

1. In a medium bowl, stir together the milk, chia seeds, and vanilla.

2. Cover and refrigerate the mixture for at least 2 hours or overnight.

3. In a blender, combine the mango, pineapple, turmeric, ginger, and honey, and blend until smooth.

4. Pour over the chia seed mixture.

5. Portion into bowls to eat immediately or into food storage containers for breakfasts during the week.

6. Before eating, add desired toppings.

breakfast burrito jars

DAIRY-FREE, GLUTEN-FREE, MAKE AHEAD, NUT-FREE,
SLOW COOKER, VEGAN

serves: 4 | serving size: 1½ cups
prep time: 10 minutes
cook time: 35 minutes to 5 hours

Don't let a busy morning get the best of your healthy eating habits. These make-ahead jars are a great way to get a filling, balanced meal each morning. Simply make one batch and portion it out into individual jars to grab and go for mornings to come.

1 cup corn kernels

1 red bell pepper, diced

½ sweet yellow onion, diced

1 (15-ounce) can pinto beans, drained and rinsed

1 cup quinoa

2 garlic cloves, minced

1 teaspoon ground cumin

1 teaspoon chili powder

Broth or water, for covering ingredients

Juice of 1 lime

Salt

1 avocado, chopped

1 handful fresh cilantro leaves

1. In a slow cooker or large pot with a lid, combine the corn, pepper, onion, beans, quinoa, garlic, cumin, and chili powder.

2. Fill with enough water or broth to cover the ingredients by about 1 inch.

3. If using a slow cooker, cook on low for about 5 hours. If cooking on the stovetop, simmer over low heat for about 30 minutes.

4. Add the lime juice and salt to taste.

5. Portion into jars.

6. Top each with the avocado and cilantro, cover, and refrigerate.

breakfast stuffed peppers

DAIRY-FREE, GLUTEN-FREE, GRAIN-FREE, MAKE AHEAD,
NUT-FREE, VEGETARIAN

serves: 4 | serving size: 1 pepper
prep time: 10 minutes | cook time: 30 minutes

Forget wraps, bread, and pitas. Peppers make a great natural vessel. This is another dish that can be adapted to whatever leftover veggies you have on hand. Also, if you're vegan, skip the egg and add chickpeas to the vegetable sauté. These peppers can be made ahead of time and eaten throughout the week.

4 bell peppers, any color, halved and seeded

2 tablespoons extra-virgin olive oil (or coconut oil), plus more for brushing peppers

2 Yukon Gold potatoes, diced

1 zucchini, diced

½ sweet yellow onion, diced

1 cup spinach

½ teaspoon dried oregano

½ teaspoon red pepper flakes

Salt

Freshly ground black pepper

4 large eggs

1. Preheat the oven to 350°F, and line a baking sheet with aluminum foil.

2. Brush the peppers with olive oil and set them on the baking sheet, then cover with foil and bake for about 10 minutes.

3. Meanwhile, in a large skillet over medium-high heat, sauté the potatoes, zucchini, and onion in 2 tablespoons of oil.

4. Once golden, after about 7 minutes, add the spinach, oregano, and red pepper flakes, and sauté until the spinach is wilted. Season to taste with salt and pepper.

5. Remove the peppers from the oven.

6. Divide the filling among each pepper, and crack 1 egg into each half.

7. Cover with foil (do not press tightly onto the peppers; leave room so the eggs don't stick).

8. Bake for 15 minutes, or until the eggs are cooked to your desired consistency. Serve or cool and refrigerate.

tempeh sausage patties

DAIRY-FREE, GLUTEN-FREE, GRAIN-FREE, MAKE AHEAD,
NUT-FREE, QUICK, VEGAN

serves: 4 | serving size: 2 patties
prep time: 10 minutes | cook time: 15 minutes

These hearty patties take care of all my breakfast sausage cravings. I love making a big batch and eating them not only for breakfast with fruit, but also over greens for lunch, drizzled with Golden Tahini Dressing (page 172).

1 (8-ounce) package tempeh

1 baked sweet potato, peeled

¼ cup dried blueberries, chopped

2 tablespoons tahini

1 tablespoon coconut aminos or tamari

1 tablespoon maple syrup

½ teaspoon dried sage

¼ teaspoon freshly ground black pepper

Salt

Coconut oil, for cooking

1. Crumble the tempeh into a large bowl and mash with the sweet potato.

2. Work in the blueberries, tahini, aminos or tamari, maple syrup, sage, and pepper, using your hands to combine everything thoroughly. Season to taste with salt.

3. Use your hands to form 8 patties with the tempeh mixture.

4. In a large skillet over medium heat, heat about a tablespoon of coconut oil.

5. Working in batches, add the patties to the skillet and cook for about 6 minutes on each side, until lightly browned. Repeat with the remaining patties, adding more oil as needed.

6. Serve or cool and refrigerate.

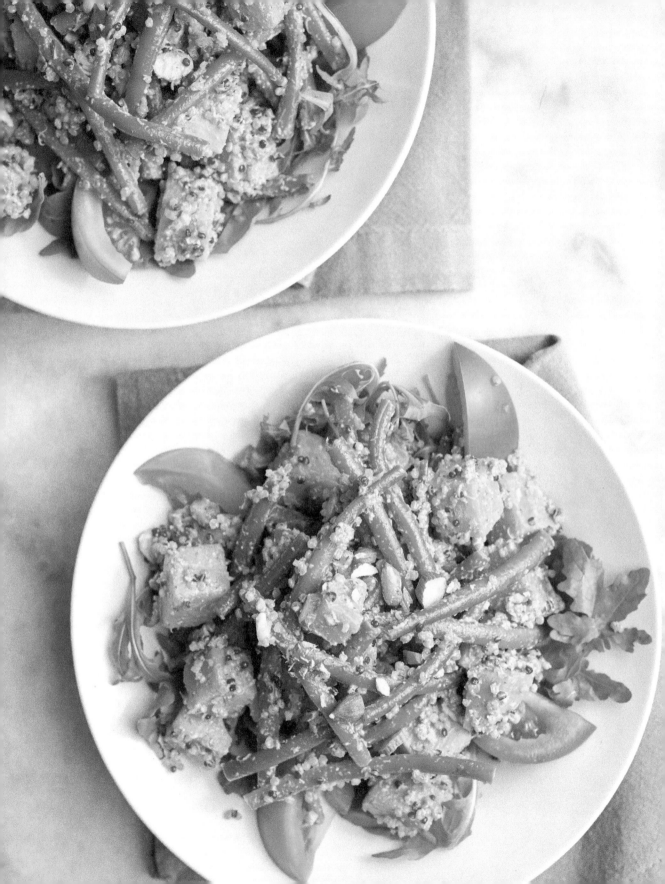

CHAPTER NINE

lunch

OPPOSITE: ALMOND & GREEN BEAN BOWL, PAGE 106

green quinoa salad

DAIRY-FREE, GLUTEN-FREE, MAKE AHEAD, QUICK, VEGAN

serves: 4 | serving size: 1½ cups
prep time: 10 minutes | cook time: n/a

This salad makes a great lunch, so prepare a big batch and portion into containers to take for lunch all week. Switch things up from day to day by adding a hard-boiled egg to one portion and extra leafy greens to another. If peas aren't in season, swap in diced cucumber.

2 cups cooked quinoa

2 avocados, chopped

1 cup fresh English peas

1 cup chopped fresh herbs (such as chives, parsley, dill, or basil)

¼ cup sunflower seeds or sliced almonds

½ cup Green Caesar Dressing (page 173)

1. In a large bowl, toss together the quinoa, avocados, peas, herbs, sunflower seeds, and Green Caesar Dressing.

2. Portion into bowls and enjoy.

peach & cucumber smash

DAIRY-FREE, GLUTEN-FREE, GRAIN-FREE, MAKE AHEAD,
NUT-FREE, QUICK, VEGAN

serves: 4 | serving size: 1½ cups
prep time: 10 minutes, plus 10 minutes to sit
cook time: n/a

Smashing cucumbers is a great technique to tenderize them, releasing more of their flavor and liquid into the dish. This meal is super refreshing on its own, but when I need a heartier dish, I toss in cooked quinoa.

2 cucumbers

¼ cup extra-virgin olive oil

½ teaspoon salt

2 peaches, sliced

1 cup shelled edamame

½ jalapeño pepper, thinly sliced

2 tablespoons white balsamic vinegar

½ teaspoon ground cumin

1. Put the cucumbers in a resealable plastic bag and press the air out.

2. Use a rolling pin to "smash" them. Use your hands to tear them apart more if needed, and place in a large bowl.

3. Drizzle the olive oil over the cucumbers, and sprinkle with the salt. Let sit for 10 minutes.

4. Add the peach slices, edamame, jalapeño, vinegar, and cumin, toss, and serve or refrigerate.

peach & pepper gazpacho

DAIRY-FREE, FREEZER-FRIENDLY, GLUTEN-FREE, GRAIN-FREE,
MAKE AHEAD, NUT-FREE, QUICK, VEGAN

serves: 4 | serving size: 1 cup
prep time: 10 minutes | cook time: n/a

News flash: Green isn't the only color of health. Deep pinks and reds are loaded with nutrients, too. This rosy-hued chilled soup is my summer meal of choice.

---

2 peaches, chopped

1 red bell pepper, chopped

1 ½ cups chopped fresh tomatoes with juices

1 shallot

¼ cup white balsamic vinegar

Juice of ½ lemon

1 tablespoon extra-virgin olive oil

Pinch salt

Ice cubes, as needed

Handful fresh basil leaves

Freshly ground black pepper

1. In a blender or food processor, combine the peaches, bell pepper, tomatoes, shallot, vinegar, lemon juice, olive oil, and salt.

2. Add a few ice cubes, and blend until smooth. Add more ice cubes as needed to reach your desired consistency or achieve a lighter flavor.

3. Pour into bowls, garnish with the fresh basil and pepper. Serve immediately, or portion into freezer-safe containers and freeze, until you need a cool, refreshing meal.

sesame veggie & quinoa bowls

DAIRY-FREE, GLUTEN-FREE, MAKE AHEAD, QUICK, VEGETARIAN

serves: 4 | serving size: 2 cups
prep time: 10 minutes | cook time: 10 minutes

I'm a big fan of grain bowls with bright colors and bold flavors. This one is so simple to toss together if you have the ingredients prepared ahead of time. This dish is why I make large batches of roasted veggies and always have a cooked grain and prepared dressing on hand.

2 cups chopped broccolini or broccoli florets

2 cups cooked quinoa

2 cups cooked diced butternut squash

1 batch Coconut-Crusted Tofu (page 163)

½ cup Golden Tahini Dressing (page 172)

1 tablespoon coconut oil

1 teaspoon toasted sesame oil

¼ cup raw pumpkin seeds

1 teaspoon sesame seeds

1. Prepare a large bowl of ice water.

2. Set a large skillet over high heat, and pour in one inch of water. Bring just to a boil, add the broccolini, and cook for 1 minute, turning as needed, until bright green. Remove from the skillet and add to the ice water to stop the cooking process and lock in that vibrant color.

3. Discard the cooking water. Add the quinoa, squash, and Coconut-Crusted Tofu to the same skillet with the coconut oil and sesame oil.

4. Cook until heated through.

5. Drain the broccoli well and add to the skillet. Stir to combine and cook just until heated.

6. Portion into bowls, sprinkle with the pumpkin seeds and sesame seeds, and serve.

moroccan carrot salad

DAIRY-FREE, GLUTEN-FREE, GRAIN-FREE, MAKE AHEAD,
QUICK, VEGETARIAN

serves: 4 | serving size: 2 cups
prep time: 15 minutes, plus 10 minutes to sit
cook time: n/a

If you come to my house for a dinner party or meet me for a picnic, chances are you'll be served this herby, sweet salad. It is a super simple dish to toss together a day in advance. Try this over brown rice, too.

½ cup extra-virgin olive oil

2 tablespoons white balsamic vinegar

2 tablespoons honey

Juice of 1 lemon

4 carrots, peeled and thinly sliced

1 cup chopped fresh herbs (dill, parsley, basil, and mint)

1 (15-ounce) can chickpeas, drained and rinsed

4 dates, pitted and chopped

½ cup roasted almonds, chopped

2 tablespoons poppy seeds

Salt

Freshly ground black pepper

1. In a medium bowl, whisk together the olive oil, vinegar, honey, and lemon juice.

2. In a large bowl, combine the carrots, herbs, chickpeas, dates, almonds, and poppy seeds, and season with salt and pepper. Pour in the dressing, and toss to coat.

3. Let sit at room temperature for 10 to 30 minutes before serving.

chickpea salad toast

DAIRY-FREE, GLUTEN-FREE, MAKE AHEAD, QUICK, VEGAN

serves: 4 | serving size: ½ cup
prep time: 10 minutes | cook time: n/a

This chickpea salad is a great substitute for egg or tuna salad and will surely become a lunch box staple. Make a batch to scoop from for the entire week.

1 teaspoon curry powder

¼ cup Golden Tahini Dressing (page 172)

1 (15-ounce) can chickpeas, drained and rinsed

1 carrot, grated

2 scallions, sliced

¼ cup chopped fresh cilantro

¼ cup golden raisins

4 slices Bird Bread (page 164)

Salad greens (optional), for serving

1. In a large bowl, stir the curry powder into the Golden Tahini Dressing.

2. Mash the chickpeas into the dressing.

3. Stir in the carrot, scallions, cilantro, and raisins.

4. Add a large scoop to each slice of toasted Bird Bread, and serve with the salad greens (if using).

warm bean & tomato toss

DAIRY-FREE, GLUTEN-FREE, GRAIN-FREE, MAKE AHEAD, QUICK, VEGAN

serves: 4 | serving size: 2 cups
prep time: 10 minutes | cook time: 5 minutes

Salads don't have to be cold. I love to toss vegetables and beans together, then serve at room temperature or warmed. It adds an element of comfort to the simple ingredients. This mix can be prepared in advance; heat just before serving.

---

1 (15-ounce) can great northern beans, drained and rinsed

2 cups chopped fresh tomatoes

2 cups chopped broccoli

½ red onion, sliced

¼ cup Kalamata olives, pitted and chopped

¼ cup chopped walnuts

¼ cup balsamic vinegar

¼ cup extra-virgin olive oil

Chopped fresh herbs, for serving (optional)

Cooked quinoa, for serving (optional)

1. In a large skillet over medium heat, combine the beans, tomatoes, broccoli, onion, olives, walnuts, vinegar, and olive oil.

2. Sauté for 5 minutes, or until the broccoli is bright green and the other ingredients are warmed through.

3. Remove from the heat. Stir in fresh herbs and quinoa (if using) before serving.

crunchy tahini toast

DAIRY-FREE, GLUTEN-FREE, MAKE AHEAD, QUICK, VEGETARIAN

serves: 4 | serving size: 1 toast
prep time: 5 minutes | cook time: 5 minutes

This toast might be my favorite lunch. It combines the hearty healthiness of fiber and complex carbohydrates, and protein provides staying power that gets me through a busy day without weighing me down. It's the contrast in textures like crisp apples with creamy tahini and flavors like sweet honey with herby parsley that make this a truly delicious bite.

4 slices Bird Bread (page 164)

Juice of 1 lemon

¼ cup tahini

1 tablespoon honey

Salt

Freshly ground black pepper

1 apple, cored and thinly sliced

1 bunch flat-leaf parsley, minced

2 tablespoons sliced almonds

1 tablespoon sesame seeds

1. Toast the Bird Bread.

2. In a small bowl, stir together the lemon juice, tahini, and honey. Season with salt and pepper to taste.

3. Cover the toast slices with the apple slices.

4. Drizzle with the tahini mixture.

5. Top with the parsley, almonds, and sesame seeds and serve.

glowing green gazpacho

DAIRY-FREE, FREEZER-FRIENDLY, GLUTEN-FREE, GRAIN-FREE,
MAKE AHEAD, NUT-FREE, QUICK, VEGAN

serves: 4 | serving size: 1 cups
prep time: 5 minutes | cook time: n/a

I call this "glowing" gazpacho because I honestly feel as though it makes my skin and mood just radiate healthy energy. Anytime you need a quick pick-me-up to boost how healthy you feel, just blend up this chilled soup.

1 lemon

1 lime

2 yellow bell peppers, chopped

2 kiwis, chopped

1 cucumber, chopped

1 cup grapes

½ cup fresh cilantro

2 cups water

1. Zest and juice the lemon and lime.

2. In a blender, combine the bell peppers, kiwis, cucumber, lemon and lime juice and zest, grapes, cilantro, and water, and blend until smooth.

3. Pour into bowls and serve chilled. This soup can also be refrigerated or frozen for later.

kale & quinoa frittata

DAIRY-FREE, GLUTEN-FREE, MAKE AHEAD, NUT-FREE, VEGETARIAN

serves: 4 to 6 | serving size: 1 slice
prep time: 10 minutes | cook time: 20 minutes

This recipe is ideal for weekly meal prep. Make the frittata, portion slices into containers, pair with fruit, and you've got healthy lunches for the week. Don't limit this frittata to the lunch box, though, as this recipe is simple enough to pull off on a busy weeknight for dinner.

---

3 tablespoons extra-virgin olive oil

1 bunch lacinato kale, finely shredded

2 garlic cloves, minced

½ teaspoon red pepper flakes (or herb of choice)

2 cups cooked quinoa

10 large eggs

1 or 2 tablespoons water

½ teaspoon salt

1. Pour the olive oil into a large, oven-safe skillet over low heat, then add the kale, garlic, and red pepper flakes. Sauté until the kale is wilted and the garlic is fragrant, 3 to 5 minutes.

2. Stir the quinoa into the kale mixture to heat through.

3. Meanwhile, crack the eggs into a large bowl. Add the water and the salt, and whisk.

4. Pour the eggs over the quinoa-kale mixture, making sure everything is evenly distributed throughout the skillet.

5. Heat the oven to broil.

6. Let the frittata cook on the stovetop for about 10 minutes, then transfer it to the oven and broil for about 4 minutes, until the eggs are set.

7. Slice and serve.

roasted orange soup

DAIRY-FREE, FREEZER-FRIENDLY, GLUTEN-FREE, GRAIN-FREE,
MAKE AHEAD, NUT-FREE, SLOW COOKER, VEGAN

serves: 4 to 6 | serving size: 1½ cups
prep time: 10 minutes | cook time: 1 hour 30 minutes

A rich, creamy bowl of warm soup is my ultimate comfort food. This bold recipe is ideal for warming the spirit and fueling the body on a chilly day. It's amazing on its own, but sometimes I use it as a base for rice, chicken, or wilted greens. If you prefer a thicker or thinner soup, use more or less liquid.

1 butternut squash, peeled, seeded, and cubed

4 oranges, quartered

4 carrots, chopped

1 white onion, chopped

3 garlic cloves

½ tablespoon cumin seeds

2 tablespoons coconut oil

3 cups vegetable broth or water

1 (14-ounce) can coconut milk

½ tablespoon ground turmeric

½ tablespoon ground ginger

Salt

Chipotle pepper flakes

1. Heat the oven to 350°F.

2. In a baking dish, mix to combine the squash, oranges, carrots, onion, garlic, and cumin seeds with the coconut oil. Roast until tender, about 1 hour, stirring occasionally. (Alternatively, you can skip the roasting and place all the ingredients in a slow cooker for 5 hours on low.)

3. Remove from the oven and allow to cool slightly.

4. Squeeze the oranges over the vegetables then discard the rinds.

5. In a blender, carefully combine the broth, coconut milk, turmeric, ginger, and roasted produce (or use an immersion blender). Do this in small batches or let cool slightly before blending.

6. Blend until creamy.

7. Season to taste with salt and chipotle flakes and serve, or transfer to storage containers and refrigerate or freeze.

lentil-stuffed potatoes

DAIRY-FREE, GLUTEN-FREE, GRAIN-FREE, MAKE AHEAD, NUT-FREE, VEGAN

serves: 4 | serving size: 1 potato
prep time: 10 minutes | cook time: 1 hour 35 minutes

Baked potatoes are another total comfort food for me. This version gets an adult makeover with leafy greens, lentils, and sun-dried tomatoes. Make a batch of these on meal prep day and refrigerate so you have meals for the week.

---

4 large potatoes (any variety)

2 tablespoons extra-virgin olive oil

1 cup arugula

1 cup spinach

2 garlic cloves, minced

½ cup cooked French green lentils

¼ cup diced sun-dried tomatoes

2 tablespoons balsamic vinegar

Salt

Freshly ground black pepper

1. Preheat the oven to 350°F.

2. Pierce the potatoes several times each with a fork. Wrap each in aluminum foil and bake until tender, about 90 minutes.

3. Meanwhile, in a large skillet over medium heat, heat the olive oil. Add the arugula, spinach, garlic, lentils, tomatoes, and vinegar, and sauté until the greens are wilted, about 5 minutes.

4. Season the lentil mixture with salt and pepper.

5. Cut each potato open, stuff with the lentil mixture, and serve.

harvest salad

DAIRY-FREE, GLUTEN-FREE, GRAIN-FREE, VEGAN

serves: 4 | serving size: ¼ of recipe
prep time: 10 minutes | cook time: 30 minutes

This salad reminds me of fall even if I'm making it in the heat of the summer or dead of winter. It has bold harvest flavors with a sweet, smoky, and spicy bite from the maple syrup and chipotle pepper. The combination of warm and cold temperatures tossed together makes it ideal for enjoying any time of year.

---

1 small butternut squash, peeled, seeded, and cubed
1 tablespoon melted coconut oil
1 tablespoon chipotle pepper flakes
1 tablespoon maple syrup
½ cup shredded red cabbage
1 apple, cored and diced
4 cups chopped kale
½ cup cooked green lentils
¼ cup raw pumpkin seeds
¼ cup chopped pecans
¼ cup dried tart cherries
½ cup Creamy Balsamic Dressing (page 174)
Salt

1. Preheat the oven to 375°F.

2. In a large bowl, toss the squash with the coconut oil, chipotle pepper flakes, and maple syrup.

3. Spread the squash on a baking sheet and roast for 20 minutes. Add the cabbage and apple to the baking sheet, tossing well. Roast for an additional 5 to 10 minutes, until the squash is tender.

4. Remove from the oven and transfer to a serving bowl. Toss with the kale, lentils, pumpkin seeds, pecans, cherries, and Creamy Balsamic Dressing. Season with salt to taste and serve.

cool & crunchy chop

DAIRY-FREE, GLUTEN-FREE, GRAIN-FREE, QUICK, VEGAN

serves: 4 | serving size: ¼ of recipe
prep time: 15 minutes | cook time: n/a

This cool, crisp salad is wonderfully refreshing, and the almond sauce adds a creamy, satisfying component. If you're eating animal ingredients, try chopped hard-boiled eggs or shredded chicken in this. Sometimes I toss in a big scoop of brown rice for a grain boost.

2 cups chopped iceberg lettuce

2 cups chopped romaine lettuce

2 large tomatoes, chopped

1 red bell pepper, seeded and diced

1 yellow bell pepper, seeded and diced

1 cup shredded carrot

2 mandarin oranges, peeled and segmented

½ cup chopped almonds or peanuts

¼ cup chopped fresh mint

2 scallions, sliced

1 tablespoon sesame seeds, for garnish (optional)

½ cup Sweet & Spicy Almond Sauce (page 177), thinned with rice vinegar or water if needed

In a large bowl, combine the lettuces, tomatoes, bell peppers, carrot, oranges, almonds, mint, scallions, and sesame seeds (if using) with the Sweet & Spicy Almond Sauce and serve.

spiced confetti rice

DAIRY-FREE, GLUTEN-FREE, MAKE AHEAD, VEGETARIAN

serves: 4 | serving size: ¼ of recipe
prep time: 10 minutes | cook time: 30 minutes

Eggplant has such a mellow, earthy flavor. In this dish, it isn't overpowered by other ingredients and there are many different textures to make the meal exciting. When I have a long or active day, this meal helps keep me satisfied for hours.

---

2 cups water
½ cup green lentils
½ cup brown basmati rice
2 tablespoons coconut oil
1 eggplant, diced
4 garlic cloves, minced
1 shallot, thinly sliced
1 teaspoon ground ginger
1 teaspoon cumin seeds
1 bunch fresh parsley, chopped
½ cup golden raisins
¼ cup Spanish peanuts
¼ cup pine nuts
2 tablespoons coconut aminos or tamari
1 tablespoon honey
1 teaspoon toasted sesame oil
Salt

1. In a medium saucepan, combine the water with the lentils and rice. Bring to a boil, then reduce the heat to low. Cover and simmer for about 30 minutes.

2. Meanwhile, in a large skillet over medium heat, heat the coconut oil until shimmering. Add the eggplant, garlic, shallot, ginger, and cumin. Stir-fry until the eggplant is tender, about 8 minutes. If the eggplant begins to brown too quickly, add a couple of tablespoons of water to the skillet.

3. Transfer the cooked eggplant, lentils, and rice to a large bowl, and combine with the parsley, raisins, peanuts, pine nuts, aminos or tamari, honey, and sesame oil.

4. Mix well, season with salt to taste, and serve.

taco salad

DAIRY-FREE, GLUTEN-FREE, GRAIN-FREE, MAKE AHEAD,
NUT-FREE, QUICK, VEGETARIAN

serves: 4 | serving size: ¼ of recipe
prep time: 10 minutes | cook time: 10 minutes

I love to make healthier whole food versions of takeout meals. This dish reminds me of my favorite taco salad, but it doesn't work against my health goals.

1 tablespoon extra-virgin olive oil

1 (15-ounce) can black beans, drained and rinsed

1 cup corn, thawed if frozen

1 teaspoon ground cumin

½ teaspoon chili powder

½ teaspoon garlic powder

4 cups chopped romaine lettuce

1 red bell pepper, diced

1 cup diced jicama or cucumber

1 cup chopped fresh tomatoes

1 bunch fresh cilantro, finely chopped

½ cup Spicy Avocado Dressing (page 170)

1. In a large skillet over medium-high heat, combine the olive oil, black beans, corn, cumin, chili powder, and garlic powder and sauté, stirring, until the corn is slightly charred, about 10 minutes. If eating right away, keep warm. If preparing ahead of time, let cool completely before adding to the cold salad.

2. Meanwhile, in a large bowl, mix together the lettuce, bell pepper, jicama, tomato, cilantro, and Spicy Avocado Dressing.

3. Top with the warm bean mix and serve.

almond & green bean bowl

DAIRY-FREE, GLUTEN-FREE, QUICK, VEGAN

serves: 4 | serving size: ¼ of recipe
prep time: 10 minutes | cook time: 10 minutes

Grain and sweet potato provide a hearty base for the bright, peppery flavors of fresh green beans, and arugula, which is enhanced even more by the addition of crunchy almonds and creamy pesto. This is a bowl that plays with texture and flavors to awaken your senses.

2 cups fresh green beans, trimmed

2 sweet potatoes, cooked and diced

1 cup cooked grains (brown rice, quinoa, farro, or wheat berries)

1 cup chopped almonds

½ cup Peppery Pesto (page 176)

2 cups arugula (optional)

1 tomato, cut into wedges (optional)

1. In a large skillet over medium heat, combine the beans, sweet potatoes, grains, almonds, and Peppery Pesto.

2. Sauté over medium heat for about 5 minutes, until the beans are bright green and everything is heated through.

3. Portion into bowls and serve over the arugula and tomato (if using).

grilled watermelon salad

DAIRY-FREE, GLUTEN-FREE, QUICK, VEGAN

serves: 4 | serving size: ¼ of recipe
prep time: 10 minutes | cook time: 5 minutes

This dish is perfect for an outdoor barbecue. It's satisfying enough to be a light summer meal but can also be an amazing side for grilled proteins. If you don't feel like grilling, use an indoor grill pan on your stovetop for the same effect.

½ small watermelon, cut into thick slices

2 cups cooked quinoa

1 avocado, peeled, pitted, and diced

4 scallions, thinly sliced

½ cup chopped almonds

¼ cup avocado oil

2 tablespoons coconut aminos or tamari

1. On the grill or in a grill pan over medium-high heat, grill the watermelon slices until lightly charred on both sides, about 4 minutes total. Remove and let cool slightly.

2. Cut the watermelon into chunks, retaining as much juice as possible.

3. In a large bowl, toss the watermelon together with the quinoa, avocado, scallions, almonds, avocado oil, and coconut aminos or tamari, mixing well for the liquids to combine.

4. Serve at room temperature.

slow cooker baked beans

DAIRY-FREE, GLUTEN-FREE, GRAIN-FREE, NUT-FREE,
SLOW COOKER, VEGAN

serves: 6 | serving size: ⅙ of recipe
prep time: 5 minutes | cook time: 6 to 8 hours

Baked beans are so comforting. I can dive into a bowl as a meal on its own, serve over sweet potatoes, or top with a creamy slaw. Slow cooker recipes like this are great for having a meal ready with very little work. No slow cooker? This can be done on the stovetop, too! Just follow the same steps, and simmer everything for about 30 minutes until the flavors have developed.

1 cup each kidney, pinto, and cannellini beans

2 (15-ounce) cans crushed tomatoes

1 sweet yellow onion, diced

¼ cup maple syrup

3 tablespoons Dijon mustard

2 tablespoons apple cider vinegar

1 tablespoon extra-virgin olive oil

1 or 2 garlic cloves

1 teaspoon red pepper flakes, plus more for seasoning

1 teaspoon smoked paprika

1 teaspoon cumin seeds

½ teaspoon ground cayenne pepper

4 cups water

Salt

1. Rinse and drain beans. In the slow cooker, combine the beans, tomatoes, onion, maple syrup, mustard, vinegar, olive oil, garlic, red pepper flakes, paprika, cumin, and cayenne with the water.

2. Cook on low for 6 to 8 hours.

3. Season with salt and red pepper flakes to taste and serve.

"cheesy" quesadillas

DAIRY-FREE, GLUTEN-FREE, QUICK, VEGAN

serves: 4 | serving size: 1 quesadilla
prep time: 10 minutes | cook time: 15 minutes

Eating whole, plant-based foods doesn't mean being restricted to raw kale and carrots. This quick meal is a favorite when I am craving a "bad" meal but refuse to give up my healthy ways. When purchasing corn tortillas, look for organic ones that contain only corn, water, and salt. If you have a panini press, use that to make your quesadillas.

1 cooked sweet potato, peeled

½ cup Spicy "Cheesy" Cashew Sauce (page 178)

½ teaspoon chipotle pepper flakes

Peppers, corn, black beans, spinach, for additional fillings (optional)

8 corn tortillas

Coconut oil, for cooking

Spicy Avocado Dressing (page 170), for serving

1. In a large bowl, mash the sweet potato with the Spicy "Cheesy" Cashew Sauce.

2. Stir in the chipotle flakes and any additional fillings (if using).

3. Spread one-quarter of the mixture onto each of 4 tortillas, and top with the remaining 4 tortillas.

4. In a large skillet over medium heat, enough coconut oil to coat the pan. Working in batches, add the quesa-dillas and cook for about 2 minutes on each side, until golden.

5. Cut into quarters, drizzle with Spicy Avocado Dressing, and serve.

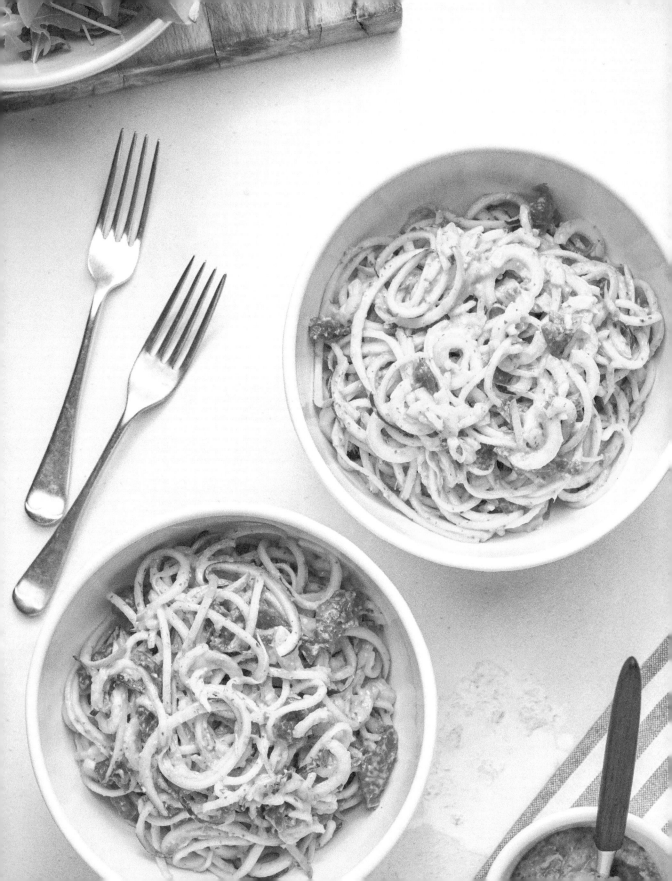

CHAPTER TEN

dinner

OPPOSITE: PESTO NON-PASTA, PAGE 124

saucy slaw bowls

DAIRY-FREE, GLUTEN-FREE, GRAIN-FREE, QUICK, VEGETARIAN

serves: 4 | serving size: ¼ of recipe
prep time: 5 minutes, plus 30 minutes to chill
cook time: n/a

This simple toss-together meal is great for days when you're in a hurry but still want to eat well. Just make the saucy slaw and serve it with whatever you have on hand. I love serving it with Coconut Rice (page 155) and Coconut-Crusted Tofu (page 163), but use your imagination and experiment with different combinations.

---

1 head green cabbage

1 red onion

1 bunch fresh cilantro, chopped

Honey-Lime Dressing (page 175)

Chopped nuts (optional)

Coconut Rice (page 155) or baked sweet potato, for serving

Coconut-Crusted Tofu (page 163), for serving

1. Finely shred the cabbage and onion into a large bowl, using a mandoline if you have one.

2. Add the cilantro and Honey-Lime Dressing. Toss well and refrigerate for 30 minutes.

3. Top with nuts (if using).

4. Serve with the Coconut Rice or sweet potatoes and Coconut-Crusted Tofu.

peach & sweet potato salad

DAIRY-FREE, GLUTEN-FREE, GRAIN-FREE, QUICK, VEGAN

serves: 4 | serving size: ¼ of recipe
prep time: 5 minutes | cook time: 5 minutes

Serving warm ingredients over cold, crisp greens is a lovely combination. It is an easy way to turn a typical salad into a complete, satisfying meal.

---

2 cooked sweet potatoes, diced

2 peaches, sliced

1 red onion, thinly sliced

½ cup mixed nuts

2 garlic cloves, peeled and crushed

¼ teaspoon ground cinnamon

½ cup Creamy Balsamic Dressing (page 174)

4 cups mixed greens

1. In a large skillet over medium heat, combine the sweet potatoes, peaches, onion, nuts, garlic, cinnamon, and Creamy Balsamic Dressing. Sauté, stirring, until golden and warm, about 5 minutes.

2. Serve over the greens.

olive & herb stuffed tomatoes

DAIRY-FREE, GLUTEN-FREE, NUT-FREE, VEGAN

serves: 4 | serving size: 1 tomato
prep time: 10 minutes | cook time: 25 minutes

During college, tuna-stuffed tomatoes were standard fare at the dining hall. This dish is my healthier, tastier adult reinvention of that collegiate staple.

---

2 cups cooked brown rice or quinoa

¼ cup extra-virgin olive oil, divided

½ cup olives, pitted and chopped

4 garlic cloves, finely chopped

¼ cup chopped fresh mint

¼ cup chopped fresh parsley

½ teaspoon red pepper flakes (optional)

1 teaspoon salt

4 large tomatoes

1. Preheat the oven to 350°F.

2. In a large bowl, mix together the rice, 2 tablespoons of olive oil, olives, garlic, mint, parsley, red pepper flakes, and salt.

3. Slice the top off each tomato. Scoop out and discard the seeds and pulp. Rub each hollowed tomato with the remaining 2 tablespoons of oil. Place in a baking dish.

4. Fill each tomato with the grain-herb mixture.

5. Bake for about 25 minutes, until tender, and serve.

loaded tabbouleh

DAIRY-FREE, GLUTEN-FREE, NUT-FREE, VEGAN

serves: 4 | serving size: 1½ cups
prep time: 10 minutes | cook time: 30 minutes

Tabbouleh is such a refreshing side dish, but I prefer to make a meal of it by adding fiber- and protein-rich lentils along with a hint of sweetness from dried fruit. This meal makes great leftovers as the flavors develop overnight, so always make enough for a second (or third) portion.

1 cup green lentils

2 cups quinoa

6 cups water

4 tomatoes, diced

1 English cucumber, diced

1 cup finely chopped flat-leaf parsley

½ cup diced red onion

½ cup dried apricots, diced

¼ cup freshly squeezed lemon juice

¼ cup chopped fresh mint

3 tablespoons extra-virgin olive oil

2 teaspoons ground allspice

1 teaspoon salt

1 teaspoon ground cumin

Freshly ground black pepper

1. In a medium pot over high heat, bring the lentils, quinoa, and water to a boil. Turn down the heat to low, cover, and simmer for 20 to 25 minutes, or until tender.

2. Drain any remaining water, and fluff the lentils and quinoa with a fork.

3. In a large bowl, combine the tomatoes, cucumber, parsley, onion, apricots, lemon juice, mint, olive oil, allspice, salt, and cumin, and season with pepper. Toss well.

4. Once the quinoa and lentils are cool, add them to the bowl, mix, and serve.

mixed grill bowls

DAIRY-FREE, GLUTEN-FREE, NUT-FREE, QUICK, VEGAN

serves: 4 | serving size: 1 cup
prep time: 10 minutes | cook time: n/a

Having prepared veggies on hand makes life so much easier. You can just pull them out, toss with a grain and greens, drizzle with dressing, and have a meal in minutes.

4 cups mixed greens

2 cups cooked brown rice (or any grain)

2 cups chopped Mixed Grilled Vegetables (page 146)

¼ cup black olives, chopped

½ cup Creamy Balsamic Dressing (page 174)

1. Place 1 cup of greens in each of four serving bowls.

2. Top each with ½ cup each of rice and Mixed Grilled Vegetables.

3. Sprinkle with the olives, drizzle with the Creamy Balsamic Dressing, and serve.

miso-mushroom stir-fry

DAIRY-FREE, GLUTEN-FREE, NUT-FREE, QUICK, VEGAN

serves: 4 | serving size: ¼ of recipe
prep time: 5 minutes | cook time: 15 minutes

I was hesitant to try miso for the first time, but honestly, now I'm addicted. The thick paste made from fermented soybeans lends an umami sensation to any dish, creating a richness I want to savor. This dish is simple to make but will replace any takeout you were used to. You can swap in any protein for the tofu.

1 tablespoon coconut oil
1 tablespoon extra-virgin olive oil
16 ounces mushrooms, sliced
1 (16-ounce) block extra-firm tofu, diced
4 garlic cloves, minced
1 tablespoon white miso paste
1 tablespoon coconut aminos
4 cups spinach
Cooked brown rice, for serving

1. In a large skillet over medium heat, heat the coconut oil and olive oil.

2. Once the oil is hot, add the mushrooms and tofu.

3. Sauté, stirring often, until the tofu is golden, about 10 minutes.

4. Stir in the garlic, miso, and aminos.

5. Add in the spinach, a handful at a time, adding more as it wilts down. Stir until all the spinach is wilted, about 5 minutes.

6. Serve over brown rice.

grilled zucchini salad

DAIRY-FREE, GLUTEN-FREE, GRAIN-FREE,
NUT-FREE, QUICK, VEGAN

serves: 4 | serving size: ¼ of recipe
prep time: 5 minutes | cook time: 10 minutes

Zucchini is likely the most versatile vegetable—well, maybe next to cauliflower, but it is definitely high on the list. Zucchini is great raw, sautéed, and grilled, in muffins, cookies, and even smoothies. Despite being a light, refreshing mix, the grilled zucchini adds a satisfying meatiness. If you are eating dairy, feta cheese is a great addition to this dish.

2 large zucchini, halved lengthwise

¼ cup extra-virgin olive oil, divided

¼ cup oil-cured olives, pitted and chopped

¼ cup chopped fresh mint

¼ cup chopped fresh parsley

2 tablespoons nutritional yeast

1 shallot, thinly sliced

Zest and juice of 1 lemon

1 teaspoon red pepper flakes

Arugula, for serving

1. Brush the zucchini halves with 2 tablespoons of olive oil. Preheat the grill, and grill the zucchini until lightly charred (or sauté in a large skillet over medium-high heat), about 10 minutes.

2. Remove from the heat. Once cool enough to touch, chop into 2-inch pieces.

3. In a large bowl, toss the remaining 2 tablespoons of oil together with the olives, mint, parsley, nutritional yeast, shallot, lemon zest and juice, and red pepper flakes. Stir in the zucchini, and serve over beds of arugula.

watermelon poke bowls

DAIRY-FREE, GLUTEN-FREE, NUT-FREE, QUICK, VEGAN

serves: 4 | serving size: ¼ of recipe
prep time: 10 minutes, plus 10 minutes to sit
cook time: n/a

Hot days are for cool, clean meals. This bowl brings me back to sunny summer days, even if I make it in the winter. Serve this dish immediately after preparing for the best results.

¼ cup rice vinegar

2 tablespoons coconut aminos

2 tablespoons tamari

Juice of 1 lime

2 teaspoons toasted sesame oil

3 cups cubed watermelon

2 cups thinly sliced cucumber

¼ cup thinly sliced scallions

¼ cup pickled ginger

2 cups cooked brown rice

Sesame seeds, for garnish

1. In a small bowl, whisk together the vinegar, coconut aminos, tamari, lime juice, and sesame oil.

2. In a large bowl, combine the watermelon, cucumber, scallions, and ginger, and pour the dressing over them.

3. Let sit for 10 minutes, tossing occasionally.

4. Serve over the rice, garnished with sesame seeds.

killer tofu kebabs

DAIRY-FREE, GLUTEN-FREE, GRAIN-FREE, MAKE AHEAD,
NUT-FREE, VEGETARIAN

serves: 4 | serving size: 2 kebabs
prep time: 15 minutes, plus an hour to marinate
cook time: 15 minutes

Going plant-based doesn't mean selling your grill on eBay. This meal is a great one when you feel like firing up the grill for outdoor barbecues and parties. You'll need eight kebab skewers (if using wooden skewers, soak them first). If you'd rather stay indoors, try a grill pan, or stir-fry all the ingredients.

---

1 (16-ounce) block extra-firm tofu, cubed (or chicken breast or mahi-mahi pieces)

2 cups pineapple chunks

2 red bell peppers, cut into large pieces

2 cups thickly sliced summer squash

1 red onion, cut into thick pieces

½ cup Honey-Lime Dressing (page 175)

Cooked brown rice or fresh greens, for serving

1. In a large resealable plastic bag or container, combine the tofu, pineapple, red peppers, squash, onion, and Honey-Lime Dressing (you can do this in two batches if needed).

2. Let the tofu, pineapple, and vegetables soak up the dressing for at least an hour. This step can be done the day before to save time.

3. Preheat the grill to high.

4. Make the kebabs by alternating pieces of vegetables, pineapple, and protein until the skewers are full.

5. Grill the kebabs for about 12 minutes (the time may vary depending on which protein you choose), rotating several times to evenly cook everything.

6. Serve over brown rice or fresh greens.

detox bowls

GLUTEN-FREE, DAIRY-FREE, QUICK, VEGAN

serves: 4 | serving size: $1/4$ of recipe
prep time: 10 minutes | cook time: 10 minutes

These bowls are mild, nourishing, and meant to soothe digestion and reduce cravings. After too much indulging or any time my body needs a reset, I turn to this dish.

---

1 (16-ounce) block extra-firm tofu, diced (or salmon)

2 tablespoons coconut or extra-virgin olive oil

2 cups cooked grains (brown rice, quinoa, or farro)

1 cup Golden Tahini Dressing (page 172)

1 cup chopped fresh parsley

2 apples, cut into thin matchsticks

½ cup raw sunflower seeds

½ cup dukkah, plus more for garnish

2 jalapeño peppers, thinly sliced

Salt

1. In a large skillet over medium heat, heat the olive oil. Sauté the tofu until golden, stirring often, about 10 minutes.

2. Portion the grains and tofu into bowls, and pour the Golden Tahini Dressing on top so it soaks into the ingredients.

3. In a medium bowl, toss the parsley, apples, sunflower seeds, dukkah, and jalapeños together before dividing among each bowl.

4. Sprinkle with more dukkah, add salt to taste, and serve.

sloppy joe lentil-stuffed peppers

DAIRY-FREE, GLUTEN-FREE, GRAIN-FREE, MAKE AHEAD, NUT-FREE, VEGAN

serves: 4 | serving size: 1 pepper
prep time: 10 minutes | cook time: 1 hour

Who doesn't love a sloppy joe? It's a classic meal that somehow signifies family and comfort. This version is different but will still provide that cozy, home-style meal feel you expect. Double this recipe because you'll want leftovers, and these reheat perfectly days later to serve over greens or with sweet potatoes.

4 large red bell peppers, halved and seeded
2 tablespoons extra-virgin olive oil, plus more for the peppers
1 sweet onion, minced
2 garlic cloves, minced
2 cups cooked black lentils
2 (15-ounce) cans crushed tomatoes
2 tablespoons balsamic vinegar
1 tablespoon maple syrup
1 teaspoon cumin seeds
½ teaspoon chili powder
½ teaspoon ground cinnamon
¼ teaspoon dried oregano
Salt
2 avocados, diced

1. Preheat the oven to 350°F.

2. Rub the peppers with olive oil and place in a baking dish.

3. In a large pot over medium heat, combine the oil and onion. Sauté for 2 minutes, stirring often. Add the garlic and cook, stirring frequently, for another minute.

4. Stir in the lentils, tomatoes, vinegar, maple syrup, cumin, chili powder, cinnamon, and oregano. Add salt to taste. Simmer, stirring often, for about 10 minutes to let the flavors develop.

5. Scoop the filling into the peppers and bake for about 45 minutes, until tender.

6. Remove from the oven, and serve. or refrigerate until ready to eat. Top with avocado before serving.

date & almond kale salad

DAIRY-FREE, GLUTEN-FREE, GRAIN-FREE, QUICK, VEGAN

serves: 4 | serving size: 1/4 of recipe
prep time: 15 minutes | cook time: n/a

Homey comfort meals with a healthy spin are great, but sometimes I just crave a kale salad. This is one of my favorites as it combines the sticky sweetness of dates with the crunch of almonds and the earthiness of fresh kale. Sometimes I like to add in brown rice or chunks of sweet potato for extra heartiness.

---

1 bunch lacinato kale, shredded

1 head broccoli, florets only, chopped

1 large apple, diced

1 cup chopped almonds

½ cup thinly sliced red onion

½ cup pitted chopped dates

½ cup sunflower seeds

1 cup Creamy Balsamic Dressing (page 174)

In a large bowl, combine the kale, broccoli, apple, almonds, onion, dates, and sunflower seeds. Toss with the Creamy Balsamic Dressing and serve.

pesto non-pasta

DAIRY-FREE, GLUTEN-FREE, GRAIN-FREE, QUICK, VEGAN

serves: 4 | serving size: ¼ of recipe
prep time: 10 minutes | cook time: 5 minutes

It's like pasta, but it's not pasta. This savory dish uses vegetables for noodles, which is a brilliant way to savor Italian flavors without consuming processed carbs. The dish itself is simple, but you can make it your own by tossing in extra Mixed Grilled Vegetables (page 146) or sardines (if including in your diet).

2 large zucchini

2 large summer squash

2 tablespoons extra-virgin olive oil

½ cup Peppery Pesto (page 176)

½ cup sun-dried tomatoes, chopped

1. Use a grater or spiralizer to turn the zucchini and squash into long strips.

2. In a large skillet over medium heat, heat the olive oil. Add the vegetable "noodles" and sauté for about 2 minutes, stirring frequently.

3. Add the Peppery Pesto and tomatoes, sauté until warmed through, about 3 minutes, and serve.

stuffed sweet potatoes

DAIRY-FREE, GLUTEN-FREE, GRAIN-FREE, MAKE AHEAD,
NUT-FREE, VEGAN

serves: 4 | serving size: 1 potato
prep time: 10 minutes | cook time: 1 hour 15 minutes

This is another one of those super comforting, homey meals turned clean. If it's stormy out, I like to make these and dig in as I watch the clouds roll in. The creaminess just makes me feel warm and safe.

---

4 medium sweet potatoes

2 cups chopped broccoli florets

1 tablespoon extra-virgin olive oil, divided

1 cup 24-Carrot Hummus (page 157)

1 teaspoon red pepper flakes

Salt

Freshly ground black pepper

1. Preheat the oven to 400°F.

2. Use a fork to poke holes in the sweet potatoes. Rub the sweet potatoes with the olive oil. Rub the rest into the broccoli and set aside. Place the sweet potatoes on a baking sheet and roast for 1 hour.

3. When the sweet potatoes are cooked, remove and let cool enough to touch. Cut a slit down the middle of each, and scoop out most of the flesh into a large bowl, leaving a shell.

4. Mix the hummus with the sweet potato flesh. Spoon the mixture back into the hollowed-out sweet potatoes.

5. Top with the broccoli, sprinkle with the red pepper flakes, season to taste with salt and pepper, and bake for another 15 minutes.

6. Cool slightly and serve.

cozy comfort soup

DAIRY-FREE, GLUTEN-FREE, GRAIN-FREE, NUT-FREE, VEGAN

serves: 4 | serving size: ¼ of recipe
prep time: 15 minutes | cook time: 25 minutes

They say soup is good for the soul. It's true. I'm not sure why, but there is no deny-ing that a bowl of steamy soup is comforting and healing. Of course, standing over a pot of soup all day likely isn't your happy place, but this soup comes together pretty quickly, so you can start feeling better in no time.

3 tablespoons extra-virgin olive oil

2 leeks (white part only), quartered and thinly sliced

4 garlic cloves, minced

3 carrots, diced

3 celery stalks, diced

2 potatoes, peeled and finely diced

6 cups vegetable broth (or chicken broth)

1 (15-ounce) can crushed tomatoes

1 teaspoon dried parsley

1 teaspoon dried oregano

1 teaspoon caraway seeds

Salt

Freshly ground black pepper

2 cups finely chopped kale or spinach (frozen works great)

½ cup frozen peas

½ cup frozen corn kernels

1. Set a large soup pot over medium heat. Pour in the olive oil, and add the leeks, garlic, carrots, celery, and potatoes. Cook, stirring frequently, for about 4 minutes, being careful to not let the garlic burn.

2. Add the broth, tomatoes, parsley, oregano, and caraway seeds, and season with salt and pepper. Reduce the heat and simmer on low, covered, for about 15 minutes.

3. Uncover the pot, add the kale, peas, and corn, and simmer for another 4 minutes.

4. Ladle into bowls, season with addi-tional salt and pepper if needed, and serve.

verde rice & beans

DAIRY-FREE, FREEZER-FRIENDLY, GLUTEN-FREE, MAKE AHEAD,
NUT-FREE, SLOW COOKER, VEGAN

serves: 4 | serving size: ¼ of recipe
prep time: 10 minutes | cook time: 2 to 6 hours

This is a fun twist on a classic burrito, but without the overprocessed tortilla and with less work. With a few minutes of dicing followed by setting a timer and pressing "on," and you'll have a meal. Once cooked, you can portion some into freezer bags to have on hand to quickly reheat anytime.

---

1 tablespoon extra-virgin olive oil

2 green bell peppers, seeded and sliced

1 yellow onion, diced

3 garlic cloves, minced

1 jalapeño pepper, sliced

1 teaspoon ground cumin

1 teaspoon ground coriander

1½ cups vegetable broth

2 (15-ounce) cans black beans, drained and rinsed

1 jar salsa verde

1 cup frozen corn kernels

1 cup brown rice

2 teaspoons chili powder

½ teaspoon salt

1 cup water

Avocado, chopped fresh cilantro, lime, yogurt (if including in your diet), for topping (optional)

1. In a large skillet over medium heat, heat the olive oil. Add the bell peppers, onion, garlic, jalapeño, cumin, and coriander, and sauté for about 3 minutes. (This step can be omitted if you're in a rush.)

2. Transfer the mixture to the slow cooker and combine with the broth, beans, salsa verde, corn, rice, chili powder, salt, and water. Stir to combine.

3. Cook for 2 hours on high or 6 hours on low.

4. Portion into bowls and serve with the toppings (if using).

falafel bowls

DAIRY-FREE, GLUTEN-FREE, GRAIN-FREE, MAKE AHEAD, VEGAN

serves: 4 | serving size: ¼ of recipe
prep time: 10 minutes | cook time: 25 minutes

Having hummus and dressing prepped in advance makes this dish a breeze. I suggest making these items on your meal prep day so that day-to-day eating is super simple. I also like saving some falafel balls to eat for snacks.

For the falafel

1 cup 24-Carrot Hummus (page 157)
½ cup almond meal
½ orange bell pepper, finely diced
¼ cup minced chives
¼ cup raw sunflower seeds
Salt
Freshly ground black pepper

For the bowls

4 cups mixed greens
1 English cucumber, diced
1 cup diced cherry tomatoes
½ cup chopped fresh parsley
1 cup Spicy Avocado Dressing (page 170)

To make the falafel

1. Preheat the oven to 350°F. Line a baking sheet with parchment paper.

2. In a large bowl, combine the 24-Carrot Hummus, almond meal, bell pepper, chives, and sunflower seeds. Use a spatula to really work the ingredients together until all the almond meal is incorporated. Season with salt and pepper to taste.

3. Use a small cookie scoop to form uniform balls of the mix. Place onto the prepared baking sheet. Bake for about 25 minutes, until golden and firm.

To make the bowls

While the falafel are baking, evenly divide the greens, cucumber, tomatoes, and parsley among 4 bowls. Top with 4 falafel each, drizzle with the Spicy Avocado Dressing, and serve.

squash bowls

DAIRY-FREE, GLUTEN-FREE, NUT-FREE, VEGAN

serves: 4 | serving size: ¼ of recipe
prep time: 10 minutes | cook time: 45 minutes

Roasting vegetables is a delicious way to turn a salad into a satisfying, warm meal by bringing out their natural sweetness. This version highlights my favorite starchy vegetable—butternut squash—in my favorite way to consume it: roasted and redolent with a smoky maple flavor.

½ butternut squash, peeled and cubed

1 cup radishes, trimmed and quartered

2 tablespoons maple syrup

1 tablespoon coconut oil

1 teaspoon smoked paprika

1 teaspoon ground cumin

1 teaspoon garlic powder

½ teaspoon salt

½ teaspoon freshly ground black pepper

2 cups cooked brown rice

2 cups arugula

2 tablespoons balsamic vinegar

Sunflower seeds, sesame seeds, and/or fresh parsley, for topping (optional)

1. Preheat the oven to 350°F.

2. In a large bowl, toss the squash and radishes with the maple syrup, coconut oil, paprika, cumin, garlic powder, salt, and pepper. Spread onto a baking sheet and roast for 45 minutes.

3. Meanwhile, in a large bowl, toss the rice, arugula, and vinegar together.

4. Divide the cooked vegetables among 4 bowls, and serve with the toppings (if using).

lentil & vegetable curry

DAIRY-FREE, FREEZER-FRIENDLY, GLUTEN-FREE, GRAIN-FREE,
MAKE AHEAD, NUT-FREE, SLOW COOKER, VEGAN

serves: 4 | serving size: ¼ of recipe
prep time: 5 minutes | cook time: 2 to 6 hours

Curry takes me back to family meals ordered out on busy weeknights. This is a much healthier, but just as flavorful, option. This meal can be made in a slow cooker or on the stovetop, and extras can be placed in freezer bags for a fast meal another night.

1 tablespoon coconut oil

2 carrots, diced

1 yellow onion, diced

1 red bell pepper, diced

1 sweet potato, diced

2 cups diced tomatoes

1 cup yellow lentils

1 (14-ounce) can coconut milk

1 cup water

1 tablespoon curry powder

1 tablespoon coconut aminos or tamari

3 garlic cloves, minced

½ teaspoon ground ginger

1 red chile pepper, sliced (optional)

Brown rice, spinach, and crushed peanuts, for serving (optional)

1. In a large skillet over medium heat, heat the coconut oil. Sauté the carrots, onion, and pepper for 5 minutes, stirring frequently. If you are in a hurry, skip this step.

2. Add the sautéed mixture to the slow cooker, along with the sweet potato, tomatoes, lentils, coconut milk, water, curry powder, coconut aminos or tamari, garlic, ginger, and red chile (if using).

3. Cook for 2 hours on high or 6 hours on low.

4. If you're not using a slow cooker, simmer in a large pot on the stovetop until tender, about 30 minutes.

5. Portion into bowls and serve with rice, spinach, and crushed peanuts (if using).

"cheesy" broccoli & rice

DAIRY-FREE, GLUTEN-FREE, VEGAN

serves: 4 | serving size: ¼ of recipe
prep time: 5 minutes | cook time: 30 minutes

Cheesy rice with vegetables diced so small they were impossible to pick out was a childhood staple for me. This version definitely strays from that classic, but in the best way, by using a nutrient-rich vegan "cheese" and nutty brown rice.

---

1 tablespoon extra-virgin olive oil

1 cup brown rice

2 cups water

1 cup diced carrots

Salt

Freshly ground black pepper

1 teaspoon garlic powder

2 cups chopped broccoli florets

1 (15-ounce) can white beans, drained and rinsed

½ cup Spicy "Cheesy" Cashew Sauce (page 178)

1. In a large skillet over medium-high heat, heat the olive oil. Toast the rice for about 2 minutes, stirring frequently.

2. Add the water, carrots, and garlic powder. Bring to a boil, then reduce the heat to a simmer, cover, and cook for 20 minutes.

3. Remove the lid and add the broccoli, beans, and Spicy "Cheesy" Cashew Sauce.

4. Continue to cook until the rice is tender, adding additional water if needed, and serve. Salt and pepper to taste.

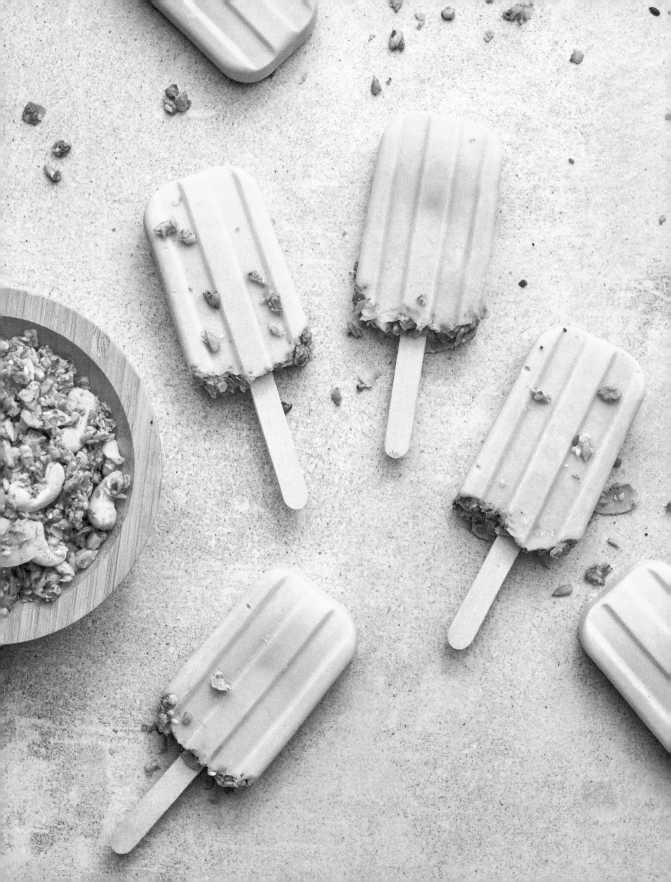

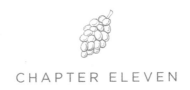

CHAPTER ELEVEN

dessert

OPPOSITE: AVOCADO POPS, PAGE 136

crunchy oat bars

GLUTEN-FREE, MAKE AHEAD, NUT-FREE, VEGETARIAN

serves: 9 | serving size: 1 bar
prep time: 10 minutes | cook time: 30 minutes

These bars are such a sweet, crispy treat. Crumble them into your yogurt or on top of cut fruit to make them more of a granola than a dessert.

Nonstick cooking spray

2 cups oats

1 cup unsweetened shredded coconut

½ teaspoons salt

¼ cup raw turbinado sugar

¼ cup flaxseed

¼ cup toasted sesame seeds

2 tablespoons psyllium powder

¾ cup (1 ½ sticks) butter

¼ cup honey

1. Preheat the oven to 350°F, and lightly grease an 11-by-7 cake pan with cooking spray.

2. In a large bowl, combine the oats, coconut, salt, sugar, flaxseed, sesame seeds, and psyllium powder.

3. In a small pan over low heat, melt the butter and honey. Add to the bowl of dry ingredients, and mix well to coat.

4. Transfer the mixture to the prepared cake pan, pressing firmly into an even layer.

5. Bake for 25 minutes, until lightly browned. Remove and let cool completely before cutting into 9 bars and serving.

banana splits

DAIRY-FREE, FREEZER-FRIENDLY, GLUTEN-FREE, GRAIN-FREE, MAKE AHEAD, VEGAN

serves: 4 | serving size: 1 cup
prep time: 10 minutes, plus 10 minutes to freeze
cook time: 5 minutes

Banana sundaes remind me of being a kid in the summer. These banana splits aren't quite as indulgent as your childhood version, but they are still delicious and make a great adult treat.

¼ cup coconut butter

1 tablespoon maple syrup

1 teaspoon vanilla extract

½ teaspoon ground cinnamon

4 bananas, halved lengthwise

¼ cup almond butter (or Super Seed & Nut Butter, page 169)

¼ cup crushed walnuts

Sea salt flakes

1. In a small pan over low heat, melt the coconut butter. Stir in the maple syrup, vanilla, and cinnamon.

2. Line a baking sheet with parchment paper, and place the banana halves on it.

3. Spread each banana half with the almond butter.

4. Sandwich the other banana halves back together.

5. Drizzle with the coconut butter mixture, and immediately sprinkle with the walnuts and salt.

6. Place in the freezer until the coconut butter mixture has hardened, about 10 minutes.

7. Take out and eat, or cover and store in the freezer until you need a treat.

avocado pops

DAIRY-FREE, FREEZER-FRIENDLY, GLUTEN-FREE, MAKE AHEAD, VEGAN

serves: 4 to 6 | serving size: 1 ice pop
prep time: 5 minutes, plus overnight to freeze and
to chill coconut milk | cook time: n/a

These aren't the ice pops I grabbed from the ice cream truck as a kid. They lack the cartoon faces drawn in food coloring and sugar to keep me running around the neighborhood for hours, but these taste so refreshing on a hot day that I don't mind the missing sugar high.

1 (14-ounce) can coconut milk, refrigerated overnight

2 avocados, pitted

2 bananas, frozen

1 cup nut milk (or yogurt, for a creamier ice pop)

Juice of 1 lime

Granola (optional)

1. Remove the coconut solids from the coconut milk can and place in the blender. Blend until creamy. Reserve the coconut water in the can.

2. Add the avocados, bananas, nut milk, coconut water, and lime juice.

3. Blend until creamy.

4. Pour into 4 to 6 ice pop molds (depending on the size of your molds), filling each three-quarters full.

5. Sprinkle granola on the top of each (if using).

6. Cover and insert ice pop sticks.

7. Freeze overnight and serve.

harvest haystacks

DAIRY-FREE, GLUTEN-FREE, MAKE AHEAD, VEGAN

serves: 12 | serving size: 2 bites
prep time: 10 minutes, plus 20 minutes to chill
cook time: 5 minutes

Sure, I eat these year-round, but they are especially delicious in autumn. Just as I don't limit them to one season, I don't limit noshing on these to dessert only; they make great snacks, too.

½ large cooked sweet potato, peeled

½ cup tahini (or nut butter)

¼ cup maple syrup

1 tablespoon coconut oil

1 teaspoon salt

1 teaspoon vanilla extract

½ teaspoon pumpkin pie spice

2 cups oats

1 cup walnuts, chopped

1 cup unsweetened shredded coconut

Dash ground cayenne pepper (optional)

1. Mash the sweet potato, but stop before you get to a purée, as some chunks are nice.

2. In a saucepan over medium heat, stir together the tahini, maple syrup, coconut oil, salt, vanilla, and pumpkin pie spice.

3. Once the mixture loosens up as it warms, stir in the sweet potato, oats, walnuts, coconut, and cayenne (if using). The mixture should be thick.

4. Line a baking sheet with parchment paper. Using a small cookie scoop, form 24 bites, and place them on the prepared baking sheet.

5. Transfer the sheet of haystacks to the refrigerator and chill until firm, about 20 minutes, before serving.

strawberry bliss bites

DAIRY-FREE, FREEZER-FRIENDLY, GLUTEN-FREE, MAKE AHEAD,
QUICK, VEGAN

serves: 7 | serving size: 2 bites
prep time: 10 minutes | cook time: n/a

These sweet, dense little balls of energy will satisfy any dessert craving. They're also easy to make and take, or save for later.

---

2 cups raw cashews

1 cup dates, pitted

1 cup freeze-dried strawberries

½ cup unsweetened shredded coconut

½ cup oats, plus extra for rolling

1 teaspoon vanilla extract

1 teaspoon salt

1. In a food processor or high-powered blender, combine the cashews, dates, strawberries, coconut, oats, vanilla, and salt.

2. Pulse until the mixture forms into a sticky mass.

3. Transfer to a large bowl, and use clean hands to tightly form 14 bite-size balls.

4. Roll the balls in the remaining oats to coat.

5. Store in the refrigerator for up to 2 weeks or for 2 months in the freezer.

vanilla-coconut shake

DAIRY-FREE, GLUTEN-FREE, GRAIN-FREE, NUT-FREE, QUICK, VEGAN

serves: 4 | serving size: 1 cup
prep time: 10 minutes | cook time: n/a

Getting a thick, creamy, sweet milkshake is one of my favorite food joys. Instead of going out, whip this healthy one up at home.

---

2 cups frozen young coconut meat

4 peeled bananas, frozen

1 cup coconut water

2 teaspoons vanilla extract

½ teaspoon ground ginger

1 cup Greek yogurt (if using dairy) or cultured coconut yogurt

1. In a blender, combine the coconut, bananas, coconut water, vanilla, ginger, and yogurt (if using), and blend until completely smooth.

2. Serve immediately.

snickerdoodle cookie dough

DAIRY-FREE, GLUTEN-FREE, GRAIN-FREE, MAKE AHEAD, NUT-FREE, VEGAN

serves: 8 | serving size: 2 tablespoons
prep time: 10 minutes, plus 2 hours to chill
cook time: n/a

There are two kinds of people in this world: Those who like cookies baked and those who would rather eat the raw batter. I am the latter. This recipe provides a healthier option to satisfy those cookie dough cravings.

---

1 (15-ounce) can chickpeas, drained and rinsed

½ cup tahini (or nut butter)

¼ cup maple syrup

1 tablespoon chia seeds

1 tablespoon flax meal

1 ½ teaspoons ground cinnamon

1 teaspoon vanilla extract

½ teaspoon salt

1. In a food processor or high-powered blender, process the chickpeas, tahini, maple syrup, chia seeds, flax meal, cinnamon, vanilla, and salt until smooth.

2. Scoop the "dough" into a sealed container, and place in the refrigerator to chill for 2 hours.

3. Eat immediately or keep refrigerated.

sesame-honey popcorn

DAIRY-FREE, GLUTEN-FREE, NUT-FREE, QUICK, VEGETARIAN

serves: 6 | serving size: 2 cups
prep time: 5 minutes | cook time: 5 minutes

Everyone likes movie night, especially when there's fresh popcorn. I am a superfan of this sweet, savory popcorn because it is satisfying without any of the guilt.

½ cup popcorn kernels

3 tablespoons coconut oil, divided

⅓ cup honey

½ tablespoon toasted sesame oil

2 tablespoons sesame seeds

Salt

Red pepper flakes (optional)

1. Line a baking sheet with parchment paper. Set aside.

2. In a large pot with a lid, combine the kernels and 1 tablespoon of coconut oil. Cover and turn the heat to high, swirling and shaking the pot every few seconds to prevent the kernels from burning. Continue this until the kernels start to pop, then let them pop until the popping slows and almost stops.

3. Carefully remove the lid and let the steam escape. Spread the popped popcorn out on the prepared baking sheet.

4. In a small saucepan over medium heat, mix the honey, the remaining 2 tablespoons of coconut oil, and the sesame oil together.

5. Allow the mixture to come to a low boil for 1 to 2 minutes, stirring occasionally.

6. Slowly drizzle the honey mixture over the popcorn. Sprinkle with the sesame seeds, salt, and red pepper flakes (if using).

7. Let cool for a couple of minutes before serving.

beany brownies

DAIRY-FREE, GLUTEN-FREE, GRAIN-FREE, MAKE AHEAD, VEGAN

serves: 9 | serving size: 1 brownie
prep time: 10 minutes, plus 15 minutes to soak
cook time: 40 minutes, plus 30 minutes to cool

Using black beans as a brownie base is a surprising way to include fiber and protein in your dessert. Don't be scared. These will not taste like beans. The flavor is rich, dense, and naturally sweet.

½ cup dates, pitted and chopped

1 (15-ounce) can black beans, drained and rinsed

½ cup almond meal

⅓ cup cacao powder

¼ cup coconut oil

2 tablespoons maple syrup

1 tablespoon flax meal mixed with 3 tablespoons water

1 teaspoon peppermint extract

½ teaspoon salt

Large handful dark chocolate chunks or cacao nibs (optional)

1. Preheat the oven to 350°F, and line an 8-by-8-inch or 9-by-9-inch baking dish with parchment paper.

2. Soak the dates in hot water for 15 minutes, until soft. Drain the water.

3. In a blender or food processor, combine the soaked dates with the beans, almond meal, cacao powder, coconut oil, maple syrup, flax mixture, peppermint extract, and salt.

4. Blend, scraping down the sides as needed to combine everything well.

5. Stir in the chocolate chunks (if using).

6. Pour the mixture into the baking dish and spread evenly.

7. Bake for 35 to 40 minutes, until a toothpick inserted into the center comes out clean.

8. Let the brownies cool completely (30 minutes or more) before cutting into 9 squares and serving. The mixture must set, and the flavors are fudgy and rich once cooled.

fruit crumble

GLUTEN-FREE, MAKE AHEAD, SLOW COOKER, VEGETARIAN

serves: 8 | serving size: 1 large scoop
prep time: 15 minutes | cook time: 2 to 3 hours

I love putting this recipe in the slow cooker and letting the house fill with the scent of fruit pie. There's very little prep to do, and using frozen fruit makes this the ultimate easy dessert.

¼ cup ghee, plus more to coat the slow cooker

4 cups fruit (chopped apples or a mix of berries)

Zest of 1 lemon

1 tablespoon freshly squeezed lemon juice

1 tablespoon flax meal

½ cup honey, divided

1 cup oats

½ cup almond meal

½ cup sliced almonds

½ cup unsweetened shredded coconut (optional)

1 teaspoon ground cinnamon

1 teaspoon ground ginger

½ teaspoon ground nutmeg

½ teaspoon salt

Greek yogurt or nut milk, for serving (optional)

1. Spread a light layer of ghee on the inside of a 6-quart slow cooker.

2. Pour the fruit into the bottom. Stir in the lemon zest, lemon juice, flax meal, and ¼ cup of honey.

3. In a large bowl, combine the oats, almond meal, almonds, coconut (if using), cinnamon, ginger, nutmeg, salt, and the remaining ¼ cup of honey. Use a fork to mix in the remaining ¼ cup ghee until the mixture is crumbly. Spread the mixture evenly over the fruit.

4. Cover and cook on high for 2 hours or on low for 3 hours.

5. Serve topped with Greek yogurt or nut milk, if desired.

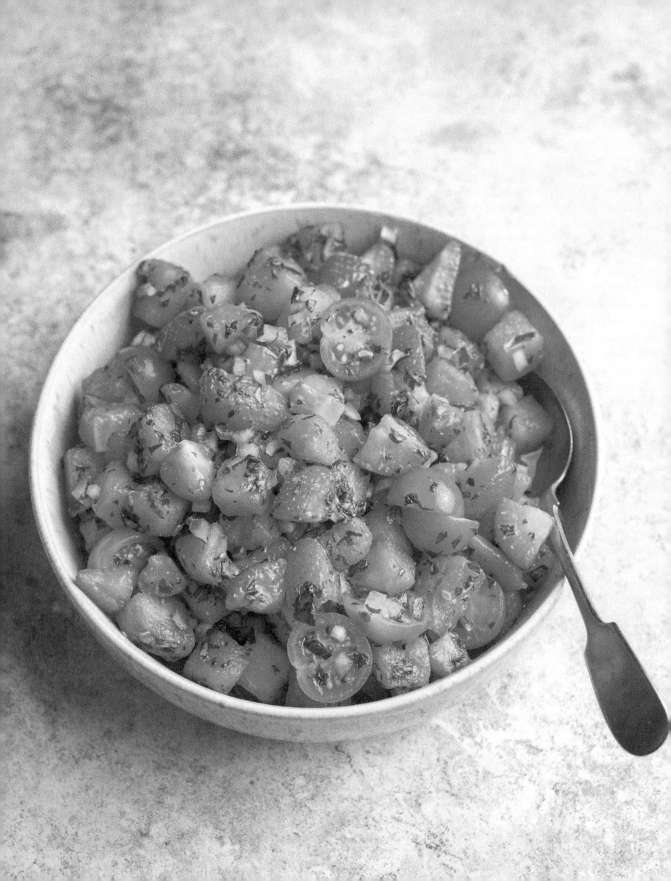

CHAPTER TWELVE

snacks & sides

OPPOSITE: WATERMELON SALSA, PAGE 147

mixed grilled vegetables

DAIRY-FREE, GLUTEN-FREE, GRAIN-FREE, MAKE AHEAD, NUT-FREE, VEGAN

serves: 4 | serving size: 1 cup
prep time: 40 minutes | cook time: 10 minutes

This blend of vegetables is a colorful, simple way to have veggies on hand for tossing into soups, salads, rice dishes, or even hummus. Try making a large batch and keeping extra around so you never run out of prepared vegetables.

For the marinade

¼ cup extra-virgin olive oil, plus more
    for seasoning
Handful fresh parsley, finely chopped
Handful chives, finely chopped
2 tablespoons balsamic vinegar
2 garlic cloves, minced

For the vegetables

2 zucchini, ends trimmed, halved lengthwise
2 summer squash, ends trimmed, halved
    lengthwise
2 red onions, cut into thick slices
1 pint cherry tomatoes
Salt
Freshly ground black pepper

To make the marinade

1. In a large bowl, mix together the olive oil, parsley, chives, vinegar, and garlic.

2. Pour into a large, resealable plastic bag. Set aside.

To make the vegetables

1. Add the zucchini, squash, onions, and tomatoes to the bag of marinade. Season with salt and pepper. Use your fingers to gently massage the marinade into the vegetables.

2. Let the bag sit for at least 30 minutes or up to 4 hours in the refrigerator.

3. Preheat the grill or grill pan on the stove to high.

4. Remove the vegetables from the marinade and grill for about 6 minutes, rotating as needed, until they start to brown.

5. Remove from the grill and, once cool enough to touch, coarsely chop.

6. Use right away or let cool and store in the refrigerator for up to several days.

watermelon salsa

DAIRY-FREE, GLUTEN-FREE, GRAIN-FREE, MAKE AHEAD, NUT-FREE, VEGAN

serves: 6 or more as a condiment | serving size: $1/3$ cup
prep time: 10 minutes, plus 30 minutes to marinate
cook time: n/a

A scoop of this salsa adds a refreshing boost to tacos, rice bowls, and grilled proteins. Personally, my favorite way to eat this is to dig right in with plantain chips.

---

3 cups diced fresh watermelon

1 cup diced fresh strawberries

1 cup cherry tomatoes, halved

½ cup minced red onion

2 tablespoons avocado oil

2 tablespoons finely chopped fresh mint

2 tablespoons finely chopped fresh basil

Juice of 1 lime

Salt

1. In a large bowl, toss to combine the watermelon, strawberries, tomatoes, onion, avocado oil, mint, basil, and lime juice. Season with salt.

2. Let sit for 30 minutes to allow the flavors to develop before serving.

3. Use immediately or store in the refrigerator for up to 3 days.

stuffed snacking dates

DAIRY-FREE, FREEZER-FRIENDLY, GLUTEN-FREE, GRAIN-FREE,
MAKE AHEAD, QUICK, VEGAN

serves: 8 | serving size: 2 dates
prep time: 15 minutes | cook time: n/a

Dates are like nature's candy. Popping a couple of these sweet and savory little treats will keep you energized for hours. I love freezing them and grabbing one or two to take with me on busy days or when traveling.

---

16 Medjool dates, pitted
½ cup Super Seed & Nut Butter (page 169)
½ cup shredded coconut

1. Slice down the side of each date, creating a "pocket."

2. Stuff each date with about ½ tablespoon of Super Seed & Nut Butter.

3. Press about ½ tablespoon of coconut onto each.

4. Consume immediately or keep chilled for later. These can be kept in the freezer for 2 months, so you can just grab a couple as needed.

smashed garlic potatoes

GLUTEN-FREE, GRAIN-FREE, NUT-FREE, VEGETARIAN

serves: 4 as a side | serving size: 4 potatoes
prep time: 10 minutes | cook time: 45 minutes

These tasty little baked potatoes are great for adding a home-style feel to any meal. Serve them with Slow Cooker Baked Beans (page 108) and roasted broccoli or slaw, or just eat them alone as a snack.

16 small potatoes (or fewer large potatoes)
½ cup ghee
8 garlic cloves, minced
2 teaspoons finely chopped fresh parsley
1 teaspoon paprika
1 teaspoon salt
½ teaspoon freshly ground black pepper

1. Preheat the oven to 375°F.

2. Pierce the potatoes several times each with a fork and place on a baking sheet.

3. Bake for about 40 minutes, until fork tender.

4. Meanwhile, in a small bowl, combine the ghee, garlic, parsley, paprika, salt, and pepper. Set aside.

5. Remove the potatoes from the oven and use a fork to press down on each and "smash" them.

6. Brush with the ghee mixture.

7. Add more salt to taste and serve.

crispy chickpeas

DAIRY-FREE, GLUTEN-FREE, GRAIN-FREE, MAKE AHEAD, NUT-FREE, VEGAN

serves: 8 as a snack | serving size: ¼ cup
prep time: 5 minutes | cook time: 30 minutes

Crispy and salty snacks typically lack everything but carbs, fat, and salt. These have all that but also fiber, plant protein, and phytonutrients. When I snack on these, I feel good about myself. If your meal needs a bit of texture or protein, just add a handful of these.

2 (15-ounce) cans chickpeas, drained and rinsed

1 tablespoon coconut oil

1 teaspoon ground turmeric

1 teaspoon ground cumin

1 teaspoon paprika

½ teaspoon salt

½ teaspoon freshly ground black pepper

1. Preheat the oven to 350°F, and line a baking sheet with parchment paper.

2. While the oven heats, pat the chickpeas dry with paper towels.

3. In a large bowl, combine the coconut oil, turmeric, cumin, paprika, salt, and pepper. Toss the chickpeas in the mixture until evenly coated.

4. Spread the chickpeas on the prepared baking sheet and roast for 30 minutes, tossing a couple of times throughout the roasting process.

5. Remove and let cool. Eat immediately or store in a lidded container in the pantry for up to 1 week.

massaged kale

DAIRY-FREE, GLUTEN-FREE, GRAIN-FREE, MAKE AHEAD, NUT-FREE,
QUICK, VEGAN

serves: 4 as a side | serving size: 1 cup
prep time: 5 minutes | cook time: n/a

This technique is a must for your whole food, plant-based eating. It is a great, simple way to boost any meal using whatever you have on hand. Kale can be a tough, hearty leafy green, which can make it tough to digest and get used to the taste. Giving it a little massage loosens up the fibers, tenderizing it while infusing it with the flavor of your favorite dressing.

4 cups shredded kale, any variety

¼ cup dressing (choose any from the recipes in this book)

1. In a large bowl, combine the kale and dressing.

2. Use clean hands to massage the dressing into the kale. Don't be timid. Really rub the kale vigorously for a couple of minutes.

3. Add to your meal, or refrigerate until needed.

golden leo latte

GLUTEN-FREE, GRAIN-FREE, MAKE AHEAD, QUICK, VEGETARIAN

serves: 4 | serving size: 1 cup
prep time: 5 minutes | cook time: 10 minutes

This latte was named for my astrological sign, Leo, whose color is gold. I think this drink is perfect for any Leo; it shines, it's bold, it's spicy, and you can depend on it to nourish your body.

4 cups nut milk

2 tablespoons almond butter

2 tablespoons maple syrup

1 tablespoon ghee

1 tablespoon grated fresh ginger (about a ½-inch piece)

1 ½ teaspoons ground turmeric

1 teaspoon vanilla extract

½ teaspoon ground cinnamon

¼ teaspoon ground cardamom

Pinch freshly ground black pepper

Pinch salt

Protein or collagen powder (optional)

1. In a small saucepan over low heat, whisk together the milk, almond butter, maple syrup, ghee, ginger, turmeric, vanilla, cinnamon, cardamom, pepper, salt, and protein powder (if using).

2. Continue whisking and simmering for about 10 minutes, to allow the ghee and almond butter to "melt" into the milk mixture and let the flavors develop.

3. Remove from the heat, whisk in the protein powder (if using), and serve.

slow-roasted red peppers

DAIRY-FREE, GLUTEN-FREE, GRAIN-FREE, MAKE AHEAD, NUT-FREE, VEGAN

serves: 4 to 8 | serving size: $\frac{1}{2}$ to 1 pepper
prep time: 5 minutes | cook time: 2 hours 15 minutes

These peppers make me think I'm in Italy. You'll want to savor each bite, because eating these is an experience in enjoying simple food. I tend to make a double batch to store in a jar and add to meals throughout the week.

4 red bell peppers
2 tablespoons extra-virgin olive oil
1 tablespoon white balsamic vinegar
1 teaspoon salt

1. Preheat the oven to broil.

2. Rub the peppers with the olive oil, vinegar, and salt.

3. Place in a baking pan and broil for about 15 minutes, turning 3 or 4 times throughout, to evenly char.

4. Once the peppers are slightly charred but not black, turn the heat off. Remove the pan, quickly cover with aluminum foil, and return to the oven to sit in the warmth for about 2 hours.

5. Take the peppers out, and once cool enough to touch, remove the skins (they should peel right off), seeds, and stems.

6. Consume immediately or add to a jar with all the juices and store in the refrigerator for up to 1 week.

crispy plantain coins

DAIRY-FREE, GLUTEN-FREE, GRAIN-FREE, MAKE AHEAD, NUT-FREE,
QUICK, VEGAN

serves: 6 | serving size: 1/6 of dish
prep time: 5 minutes | cook time: 25 minutes

Forget the chips and pass the plantains. These starchy, crispy bites are perfect to dip into hummus or guacamole, or even to crumble up and use as a healthier, whole food alternative to bread crumb coating.

---

4 green plantains

2 tablespoons melted coconut oil

½ teaspoon ground allspice

½ teaspoon ground ginger

½ teaspoon ground nutmeg

½ teaspoon ground cinnamon

Zest of 1 lime

Salt

1. Preheat the oven to 400°F, and line a baking sheet with parchment paper.

2. Chop off both ends of each plantain, and carefully slice open the thick peel and remove it.

3. Slice the peeled plantains into thin, even rounds.

4. In a large bowl, mix together the coconut oil, allspice, ginger, nutmeg, and cinnamon. Add the plantain slices, and use your fingers to gently coat.

5. Lay the slices on the prepared baking sheet and bake for 20 to 25 minutes, until crispy, flipping once.

6. Remove from the oven and sprinkle with the lime zest and salt to taste.

7. Consume right away or stash in the pantry for up to 3 days.

coconut rice

DAIRY-FREE, GLUTEN-FREE, MAKE AHEAD, NUT-FREE, QUICK, VEGAN

serves: 4 | serving size: ⅓ cup
prep time: 5 minutes | cook time: 25 minutes

Rice can get boring, but this version has some tropical flair to keep things interesting. I always make a big batch of this brown rice and keep it around to add scoops to soups or salads or to serve as a side dish to veggies and proteins.

---

1 cup brown jasmine or basmati rice
⅓ cup full-fat coconut milk
1 cup water
¾ teaspoon salt
Zest and juice of 2 limes
2 tablespoons finely chopped fresh cilantro

Rice cooker method

1. Rinse the rice several times, and transfer to a rice cooker.

2. Add the coconut milk, water, and salt, stir, and cook according to the appliance's instructions until tender.

3. Stir in the lime zest and juice and the cilantro and serve.

Stovetop method

1. Rinse the rice several times, and transfer to a small saucepan. Add the coconut milk, water, and salt. Stir.

2. Bring to a boil.

3. Reduce the heat to a simmer, cover the pot, and cook for about 15 minutes, until the water has been absorbed. Fluff the rice with a fork. Turn off the heat and let the rice sit, covered, for about 5 minutes.

4. Stir in the lime zest and juice and the cilantro and serve.

fruit & nut salad

GLUTEN-FREE, GRAIN-FREE, MAKE AHEAD, QUICK, VEGETARIAN

serves: 4 | serving size: 1 cup
prep time: 5 minutes | cook time: n/a

Snacks should fuel you up between meals, and this one won't disappoint. It's simple, can be made ahead, and provides healthy carbohydrates from the fruit and protein from the yogurt and nuts.

½ teaspoon ground cinnamon

½ teaspoon almond extract

1 cup Greek yogurt

4 cups assorted diced fruit (berries, grapes, and/or peaches)

½ cup chopped nuts (pecans, almonds, and/or walnuts)

2 tablespoons poppy seeds

2 tablespoons hemp seeds

1. In a large bowl, mix the cinnamon and almond extract into the yogurt.

2. Stir in the fruit, nuts, poppy seeds, and hemp seeds and serve.

24-carrot hummus

DAIRY-FREE, GLUTEN-FREE, GRAIN-FREE, MAKE AHEAD, NUT-FREE, VEGAN

serves: 6 to 9 | serving size: 2 tablespoons
prep time: 15 minutes | cook time: 20 minutes

Hummus is my everything. It's creamy, filling, and so versatile. Seriously, I spread it on sandwiches, dip my veggies in it, and even add a scoop to salads. This one strays from traditional plain hummus by using naturally sweet carrots for a flavor, color, and nutrition boost.

---

2 cups chopped carrots

¼ cup plus 2 tablespoons extra-virgin olive oil, divided

4 garlic cloves, peeled

½ teaspoon paprika

½ teaspoon ground cumin

⅛ teaspoon ground cayenne pepper

½ teaspoon salt

1 (15-ounce) can chickpeas, drained and rinsed

¼ cup chopped fresh parsley

2 tablespoons freshly squeezed lemon juice

1 tablespoon tahini

1. Preheat the oven to 400°F.

2. In a large bowl, toss the carrots with 2 tablespoons of olive oil and the garlic, paprika, cumin, cayenne, and salt.

3. Spread onto a baking sheet and roast for about 20 minutes, until tender.

4. Remove and allow to cool slightly.

5. Once cooled, place the carrot mixture in a food processor or high-powered blender with the chickpeas, parsley, lemon juice, and tahini. Pulse while drizzling in the remaining ¼ cup of oil. Purée until smooth.

6. Serve immediately, or store for up to 1 week in the refrigerator.

sweet, spicy & savory nuts

GLUTEN-FREE, GRAIN-FREE, MAKE AHEAD, QUICK, VEGETARIAN

serves: 8 | serving size: ¼ cup
prep time: 5 minutes | cook time: 10 minutes

I love to make these before having guests over because they provide a great snack or appetizer for a crowd. They also fill the house with a delicious, irresistible scent.

2 tablespoons ghee

1 shallot, minced

2 tablespoons minced fresh rosemary

2 cups raw mixed nuts (such as almonds, cashews, and Brazil nuts)

½ cup raw pumpkin seeds

¼ cup maple syrup

½ teaspoon salt

Pinch ground cayenne pepper

1. In a medium skillet over medium heat, melt the ghee. Cook the shallots and rosemary for about 5 minutes, stirring frequently.

2. Add the nuts and pumpkin seeds to the pan. Stir frequently until the nuts begin to get slightly toasted and fragrant.

3. Add the maple syrup and stir to coat.

4. Remove from the heat and season with the salt and cayenne.

5. Consume immediately, or, once completely cooled, cover and save for later.

energizing trail mix

DAIRY-FREE, GLUTEN-FREE, GRAIN-FREE, MAKE AHEAD, QUICK, VEGAN

serves: 16 | serving size: ¼ cup
prep time: 5 minutes | cook time: n/a

Snacks are the best when there is no real work involved, and you can just grab and go. This mix is just that. Toss everything into a large bag or jar, and keep it around for when cravings hit.

1 cup banana chips
¾ cup peanuts
¾ cup almonds
½ cup raw pumpkin seeds
½ cup dried goji berries
½ cup chopped dried apricots
½ cup unsweetened coconut flakes

1. Slightly break up the banana chips.

2. In a large bowl, toss together the banana chips, peanuts, almonds, pumpkin seeds, goji berries, apricots, and coconut flakes.

3. Store in an airtight container in the pantry.

creamed corn

DAIRY-FREE, GLUTEN-FREE, NUT-FREE, QUICK, VEGAN

serves: 4 | serving size: ¼ cup
prep time: 5 minutes | cook time: 10 minutes

As a kid I wanted nothing to do with creamed corn on my plate. It was bland, thick, and flavorless. This recipe will make you a creamed corn lover. It's bright and fresh while remaining comforting and creamy.

1 tablespoon coconut oil

½ cup sliced scallions

1 teaspoon cumin seeds

The kernels from 4 ears of corn (or 3 cups frozen corn if not in season)

1 (14-ounce) can coconut milk

2 teaspoons coconut aminos or tamari

Salt

½ cup chopped fresh cilantro

Chile peppers, sliced, or chipotle pepper flakes, for topping (optional)

1. In a large skillet over medium heat, heat the coconut oil. Add the scallion and cumin seeds, and sauté for about 2 minutes.

2. Add the corn, coconut milk, and aminos or tamari. Reduce the heat to low and cook, stirring occasionally, for 8 to 10 minutes, until the liquid begins to thicken.

3. Remove from the heat, season with salt to taste, and top with the cilantro and chile peppers (if using) before serving.

cocoa-cashew latte

DAIRY-FREE, GLUTEN-FREE, GRAIN-FREE, MAKE AHEAD, QUICK, VEGAN

serves: 4 | serving size: 1 cup
prep time: 10 minutes | cook time: n/a

Are you a caffeine addict? I am. Nothing satisfies me and perks me up for the day like a strong espresso beverage. Of course, many coffee drinks are loaded with inflammatory ingredients like fake flavors and sugar. This version is satisfying, quick, and delicious.

---

1 cup raw cashews (for a creamier texture, soak in water up to 8 hours, drain, and rinse before using)

3 cups water

2 cups brewed coffee or 4 to 8 shots espresso

4 dates

1 tablespoon cacao powder

1 teaspoon vanilla extract

⅛ teaspoon ground cinnamon

1. In a blender, blend the cashews and water until the "milk" is smooth and frothy.

2. Place a nut milk bag or cheese-cloth over a large bowl, and pour the blended mixture into it. Return the strained liquid to the blender. The cashew pulp can be stored in the refrigerator and used in desserts or for baking.

3. Add the coffee, dates, cacao powder, vanilla, and cinnamon to the blender, and blend until well mixed.

4. Serve frothy and chilled straight from the blender (at this point you can store any extra in a jar in the refrigerator for use the next day), or add to a saucepan and simmer until heated through, if you want a warm beverage.

fitness fried rice

DAIRY-FREE, GLUTEN-FREE, MAKE AHEAD, NUT-FREE, QUICK, VEGAN

serves: 4 | serving size: 1 cup
prep time: 5 minutes | cook time: 10 minutes

Fried rice is a takeout standard. Sure, it requires a little more effort to make your own, but in the time it takes you to place an order, go pick it up, and get back home, you could have prepared this nutritious version instead. Eat this alone, use as a side dish, or toss in eggs or tofu for a more substantial meal.

---

1 tablespoon extra-virgin olive oil or coconut oil

1 red onion, diced

3 garlic cloves, minced

2 cups cooked brown rice

1 cup frozen shelled edamame

½ cup sunflower seeds

2 tablespoons sesame seeds

2 tablespoons tamari

1 teaspoon Chinese five-spice powder

1 teaspoon toasted sesame oil

1. In a large skillet over medium-high heat, heat the olive oil. Sauté the onion until just tender, about 3 minutes. Add the garlic, and cook for an additional minute.

2. Add the rice, edamame, sunflower seeds, sesame seeds, tamari, five-spice powder, and sesame oil, stirring well to combine and evenly distribute the seasonings. Sauté until heated through.

3. If crispy rice is desired, turn the heat to high and cook for an extra 2 minutes without stirring.

4. Remove from the heat and serve, or let cool and store in the refrigerator for up to 5 days.

coconut-crusted tofu

DAIRY-FREE, GLUTEN-FREE, GRAIN-FREE, MAKE AHEAD, VEGAN

serves: 4 | serving size: ½ block
prep time: 10 minutes | cook time: 30 minutes

I have to admit, adding tofu to my diet took a little trial and error before I started liking it. Now I'm hooked. This is a fun way to add tofu to your meals, especially if you're not a tofu superfan. Sometimes I make these just to snack on, but other times I chop up the crusted slabs to toss into rice or salads.

2 (16-ounce) blocks extra-firm tofu

1 (14-ounce) can coconut milk

2 tablespoons nut butter

2 tablespoons rice vinegar

1 tablespoon tamari

1 tablespoon grated fresh ginger, or
  1 teaspoon dried

1 tablespoon maple syrup

1 cup unsweetened shredded coconut

½ cup flax meal

½ teaspoon ground turmeric

1. Preheat the oven to 350°F.

2. Slice each block of tofu into 4 thick slabs. Gently prick each slab several times with a fork.

3. In a large bowl, whisk together the coconut milk, nut butter, vinegar, tamari, ginger, and maple syrup.

4. Let the tofu slabs soak in the mixture for about 5 minutes, turning to coat if necessary.

5. In a separate large bowl, combine the coconut, flax, and turmeric.

6. Line a baking sheet with parchment paper.

7. Take one slab of tofu and press each side into the coconut coating. Transfer to the prepared baking sheet. Repeat until each slab is coated.

8. Bake for 30 minutes, until golden brown.

9. Use right away or let cool and store in the refrigerator for up to 1 week.

bird bread

DAIRY-FREE, GLUTEN-FREE, MAKE AHEAD, VEGAN

serves: 8 | serving size: ⅛ of loaf
prep time: 10 minutes, plus 2 hours to rest
cook time: 2 hours 30 minutes

The name says it all. This is a dense loaf that, prior to being baked, resembles a bowl of birdseed. But don't let that scare you off. The finished product is filling, nutrient rich, and delicious. While the total time is long due to the soaking and baking, the actual work required is minimal.

---

1 ½ cups oats

1 cup raw sunflower seeds

½ cup flaxseed

¼ cup raw almonds, chopped

¼ cup psyllium powder

2 tablespoons raisins

2 tablespoons chia seeds

1 teaspoon caraway seeds

1 teaspoon salt

1 ½ cups warm water

2 tablespoons coconut oil, melted

2 tablespoons maple syrup

Zest and juice of ½ orange

¼ cup chopped pitted green olives

1. In a large bowl, mix to combine the oats, sunflower seeds, flaxseed, almonds, psyllium powder, raisins, chia seeds, caraway seeds, and salt.

2. In a separate large bowl, whisk together the water, coconut oil, maple syrup, orange zest, and orange juice.

3. Pour the wet mixture over the dry ingredients, add the olives, and mix to thoroughly combine. The mixture will be thick.

4. Cover and let sit for 1 hour. Give the mixture a stir. If it is too thick to stir, add a couple tablespoons of water and stir again. Cover again and let sit for an additional hour.

5. Preheat the oven to 350°F, and line a loaf pan with parchment paper.

6. Transfer the oat mixture into the loaf pan. Press the mixture firmly down into the pan.

7. Bake for 1 hour and 30 minutes. Turn the oven off, remove the loaf from the pan (carefully), peel off the parchment paper, and return the loaf to the oven for 1 hour to continue to dry out.

8. Cut into 8 slices and enjoy immediately. Wrap any leftovers in aluminum foil or plastic wrap and store in the refrigerator for up to one week.

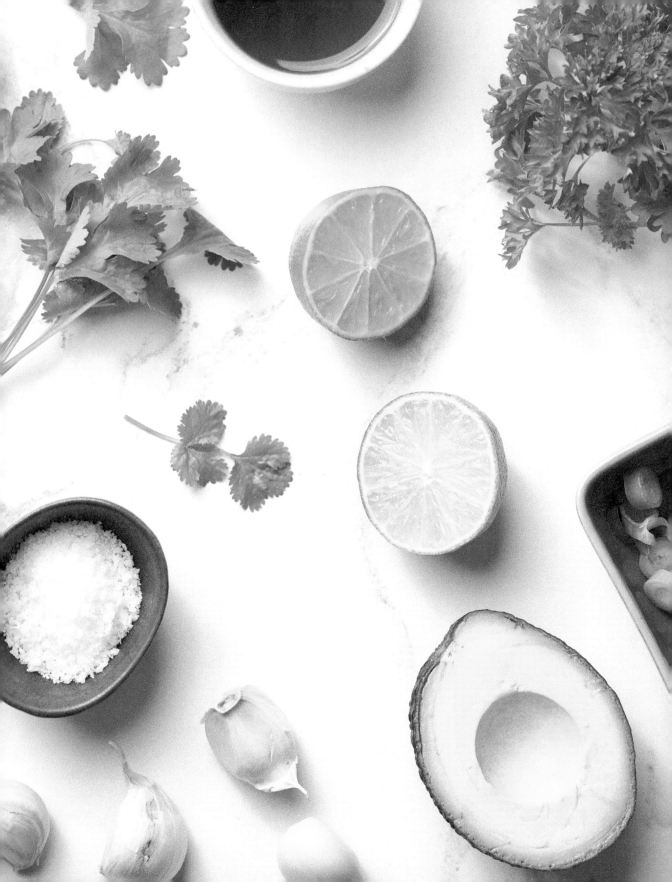

CHAPTER THIRTEEN

basics, sauces
& condiments

almond oat milk

DAIRY-FREE, GLUTEN-FREE, MAKE AHEAD, VEGAN

serves: 6 | serving size: 1 cup
prep time: 5 minutes, plus overnight to soak
cook time: n/a

Buying plant-based milk is fine, but it can be difficult to sort through the labels to find a brand that is all natural and not loaded with additives. I say, try making your own because it is pretty simple and honestly tastes so much better than a store-bought version. By adding ingredients like vanilla, maple, spirulina, cinnamon, cacao, espresso, etc., you can have fun making your own healthy varieties.

1 cup rolled oats
1 cup raw almonds
7 cups water
6 dates, pitted
1 teaspoon vanilla extract (optional)

1. Put the oats and almonds in a large container (they will expand a bit) and cover with water.

2. Cover the container and place in the refrigerator to soak overnight.

3. Drain and rinse thoroughly.

4. Transfer the soaked mixture to a blender, and add the water, dates, and vanilla (if using).

5. Blend for about 2 minutes, until well combined.

6. Place a nut milk bag or cheesecloth over a large bowl, and pour the blended mixture into it.

7. Use your hands to squeeze the mixture in the nut bag, letting the liquid drain into the bowl.

8. Transfer to a sealable container and store in the refrigerator for up to 1 week.

super seed & nut butter

DAIRY-FREE, GLUTEN-FREE, GRAIN-FREE, MAKE AHEAD, QUICK, VEGAN

serves: 16 | serving size: 2 tablespoons
prep time: 5 minutes | cook time: n/a

I can't get enough of this thick, creamy, salty spread. I add it to toast, collard wraps, and smoothies, and I even use it for sauces like the Sweet & Spicy Almond Sauce (page 177). As soon as I run out of a jar, I make another batch immediately.

1 cup raw almonds

1 cup raw sunflower seeds

½ cup raw cashews

½ teaspoon coconut oil

2 tablespoons maple syrup

1 tablespoon chia seeds

1 tablespoon flax meal

1 tablespoon hemp seeds

¼ cup raw pumpkin seeds

1 teaspoon salt

Ground cinnamon or cardamom or vanilla extract (optional)

1. Preheat the oven to 325°F, and line a baking sheet with parchment paper.

2. In a large bowl, toss the almonds, sunflower seeds, and cashews with the coconut oil and maple syrup.

3. Spread the mixture onto the prepared baking sheet.

4. Roast for about 10 minutes, stirring occasionally to prevent burning. Remove and let cool slightly. While still warm (but not hot!), transfer the mixture to a food processor or high-powered blender and pulse until the nuts begin to break down.

5. Add the chia seeds, flax meal, hemp seeds, pumpkin seeds, and salt.

6. Add cinnamon, cardamom or vanilla (if using).

7. Continue pulsing, stopping to scrape down the sides until a paste begins to form.

8. Transfer to a jar and store for up to 1 week in your pantry or 3 weeks in the refrigerator.

spicy avocado dressing

DAIRY-FREE, GLUTEN-FREE, GRAIN-FREE, MAKE AHEAD,
NUT-FREE, QUICK, VEGAN

serves: 10 | serving size: 2 tablespoons
prep time: 5 minutes | cook time: n/a

This dressing is like adding a layer of nutrient-rich, vibrant guac to your tacos, bowls, and salads. When I have an avocado that is getting a bit too ripe, I blend up this dressing to extend its lifespan and add an avocado-y kick to all my meals.

¼ cup avocado oil

½ avocado, peeled and pitted

1 cup chopped fresh parsley

1 cup chopped fresh cilantro

1 jalapeño pepper

2 scallions, chopped

4 garlic cloves

Juice of 1 lime

Salt

Water, if needed

1. In a blender, combine the avocado oil, avocado, parsley, cilantro, jalapeño, scallions, garlic, and lime juice, and season with salt. Blend until it reaches your desired consistency, adding water if necessary.

2. Store leftovers in the refrigerator for up to 1 week.

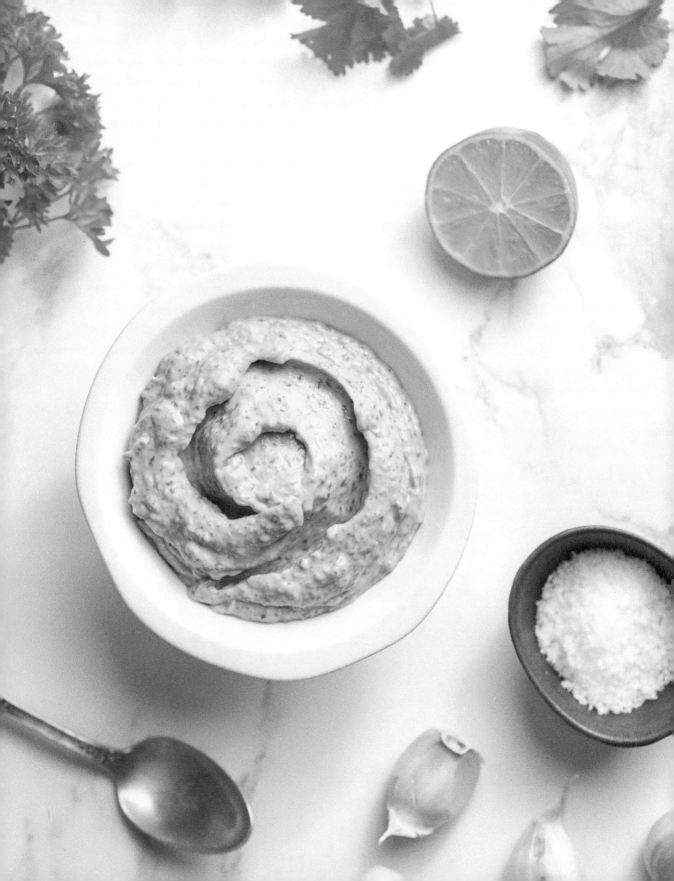

golden tahini dressing

DAIRY-FREE, GLUTEN-FREE, GRAIN-FREE, MAKE AHEAD,
NUT-FREE, QUICK, VEGAN

serves: 4 | serving size: just over ⅓ cup
prep time: 5 minutes | cook time: n/a

Turn anything to gold with this recipe! This dressing will provide a mild, creamy flavor and add a punch of bright golden color to any salad or grain bowl.

½ cup water, plus more if needed

¼ cup tahini

3 tablespoons apple cider vinegar

2 tablespoons coconut aminos

2 garlic cloves

1 tablespoon maple syrup

1 tablespoon nutritional yeast

1 teaspoon ground turmeric

¼ teaspoon freshly ground black pepper

1. In a blender, combine the water, tahini, vinegar, coconut aminos, garlic, maple syrup, nutritional yeast, turmeric, and pepper, and blend until smooth.

2. Add more water if the dressing is too thick.

3. Drizzle over salads and grain bowls.

4. Store in the refrigerator for up to 1 week.

green caesar dressing

DAIRY-FREE, GLUTEN-FREE, GRAIN-FREE, MAKE AHEAD, QUICK, VEGAN

serves: 10 | serving size: 2 tablespoons
prep time: 5 minutes | cook time: n/a

The bold, bright flavors in this green Caesar will provide a punch of flavor to any dish. Drizzle it liberally on anything and everything.

½ cup raw almonds

½ cup avocado oil

¼ cup chopped fresh parsley

7 garlic cloves

3 scallions, chopped

¼ cup white balsamic vinegar

1 shallot

Juice of 1 lemon

½ teaspoon hemp seeds

½ teaspoon salt

½ teaspoon freshly ground black pepper

½ teaspoon spirulina powder (optional)

Water, if needed

1. In a blender, combine the almonds, avocado oil, parsley, garlic, scallions, vinegar, shallot, lemon juice, hemp seeds, salt, pepper, and spirulina powder (if using). Blend until it reaches your desired consistency, adding water if necessary.

2. Store leftovers in the refrigerator for up to 1 week.

creamy balsamic dressing

DAIRY-FREE, GLUTEN-FREE, GRAIN-FREE, MAKE AHEAD, QUICK, VEGAN

serves: 10 | serving size: 2 tablespoons
prep time: 5 minutes | cook time: n/a

Balsamic and oil go well on almost anything, but I enjoy a creamy texture in my dressings. This version is great for when you want a classic taste with a little extra heft that can stand up to bold textures like potatoes, kale, and apples.

½ cup walnut oil or extra-virgin olive oil

½ cup balsamic vinegar

2 garlic cloves

2 tablespoons tahini

1 tablespoon fresh rosemary

Water, for thinning (optional)

Salt

Freshly ground black pepper

1. In a blender, combine the walnut oil, vinegar, garlic, tahini, and rosemary. Blend until the rosemary is finely chopped and the dressing is thick and creamy.

2. Add water to the blender if you desire a thinner consistency.

3. Use immediately, or store in the refrigerator for up to 1 week. Shake well before using.

honey-lime dressing

DAIRY-FREE, GLUTEN-FREE, GRAIN-FREE, MAKE AHEAD,
NUT-FREE, QUICK, VEGETARIAN

serves: 8 | serving size: 3 tablespoons
prep time: 5 minutes | cook time: n/a

This dressing is a simple way to jazz up vegetables or salads, or use it as a marinade for tofu, fish, and poultry. Make it in advance and have it on hand for when your meal needs a little bite.

½ cup fresh cilantro leaves

¼ cup avocado oil (or extra-virgin olive oil)

Juice of 2 limes

¼ cup honey

2 garlic cloves, minced

1 teaspoon salt

Sliced jalapeño (optional)

1. In a medium bowl or jar, whisk to combine the cilantro, avocado oil, lime juice, honey, garlic, salt, and jalapeño (if using).

2. Use immediately or store in a sealed jar in the refrigerator for up to 5 days.

peppery pesto

DAIRY-FREE, GLUTEN-FREE, GRAIN-FREE, MAKE AHEAD, QUICK, VEGAN

serves: 4 | serving size: 2 tablespoons
prep time: 5 minutes | cook time: n/a

I love pesto for its bright green hue and use of fresh herbs; however, traditional pestos feel heavy. This sauce is creamy because of the avocado and packs a peppery punch from the arugula.

½ cup fresh basil

½ cup arugula

1 avocado, pitted and peeled

½ cup raw cashews

¼ cup extra-virgin olive oil

2 garlic cloves, peeled

2 tablespoons freshly squeezed lemon juice

¼ teaspoon salt

¼ teaspoon freshly ground black pepper

Red pepper flakes (optional)

1. In a food processor or blender, combine the basil, arugula, avocado, cashews, olive oil, garlic, lemon juice, salt, pepper, and red pepper flakes (if using).

2. Blend for about 5 minutes, until the mixture forms a loose paste.

3. This pesto is best consumed immediately, although it can be refrigerated for up to 6 days.

sweet & spicy almond sauce

DAIRY-FREE, GLUTEN-FREE, GRAIN-FREE, MAKE AHEAD, QUICK, VEGAN

serves: 6 | serving size: 2 tablespoons
prep time: 5 minutes | cook time: n/a

I really love a good sauce. Any meal of whole, plant-based food can become more interesting when topped with a flavorful sauce. This is one of my go-tos because it can be made in minutes using simple ingredients I typically have on hand and is a great addition to any grain, salad, or protein.

½-inch piece ginger

½ cup almond butter (or Super Seed & Nut Butter, page 169)

1 tablespoon rice vinegar

1 tablespoon freshly squeezed lime juice

1 tablespoon maple syrup

Pinch ground cayenne pepper

Pinch salt

¼ cup water, as needed

1. In a blender or food processor, pulse the ginger until chopped.

2. Add the almond butter, vinegar, lime juice, maple syrup, cayenne, and salt, and pulse until smooth.

3. Slowly add the water to thin the sauce to your desired consistency.

4. Store in the refrigerator for up to 1 week.

spicy "cheesy" cashew sauce

DAIRY-FREE, GLUTEN-FREE, GRAIN-FREE, MAKE AHEAD, VEGAN

serves: 8 | serving size: 2 tablespoons
prep time: 5 minutes, plus 12 hours to soak
cook time: n/a

Going plant based means making some sacrifices, like giving up cheese. Luckily, this cashew-based "cheese" sauce is a great replacement in terms of taste and nutrients

---

1 cup raw cashews

½ cup water

¼ cup nutritional yeast

2 garlic cloves

2 teaspoons onion flakes

1 teaspoon ground turmeric

1 teaspoon chipotle pepper flakes, plus more if desired

Salt

1. Put the cashews in a large jar, and cover with cold water. Cover and let soak in the refrigerator for at least 12 hours and up to 24.

2. Rinse and drain the cashews.

3. Transfer to a blender and add the water, nutritional yeast, garlic, onion flakes, turmeric, and pepper flakes.

4. Blend until smooth and creamy, adding more water if the mixture is too thick.

5. Add more pepper flakes, if desired, and salt to taste.

6. Store in the refrigerator for up to 1 week.

quickie raspberry jam

DAIRY-FREE, GLUTEN-FREE, GRAIN-FREE, NUT-FREE, MAKE AHEAD, VEGAN

serves: 8 | serving size: 2 tablespoons
prep time: 5 minutes, plus overnight to soak
cook time: n/a

I am addicted to raspberries. They are hands down my favorite fruit. This jam is an excellent way to add raspberry flavor (naturally) to your day. I stir it into oats, scoop it onto eggs, and even shake it into nut milk for a quick "smoothie."

3 cups raspberries

2 tablespoons chia seeds

2 tablespoons maple syrup

1 tablespoon flaxseed meal

1 tablespoon freshly squeezed lemon juice

1 teaspoon ground cardamom

1. In a large bowl, mash the berries with a fork.

2. Stir in the chia seeds, maple syrup, flaxseed meal, lemon juice, and cardamom.

3. Let sit overnight in the refrigerator to allow the flax and chia to bind and thicken.

4. Use immediately or keep refrigerated for up to 1 week.

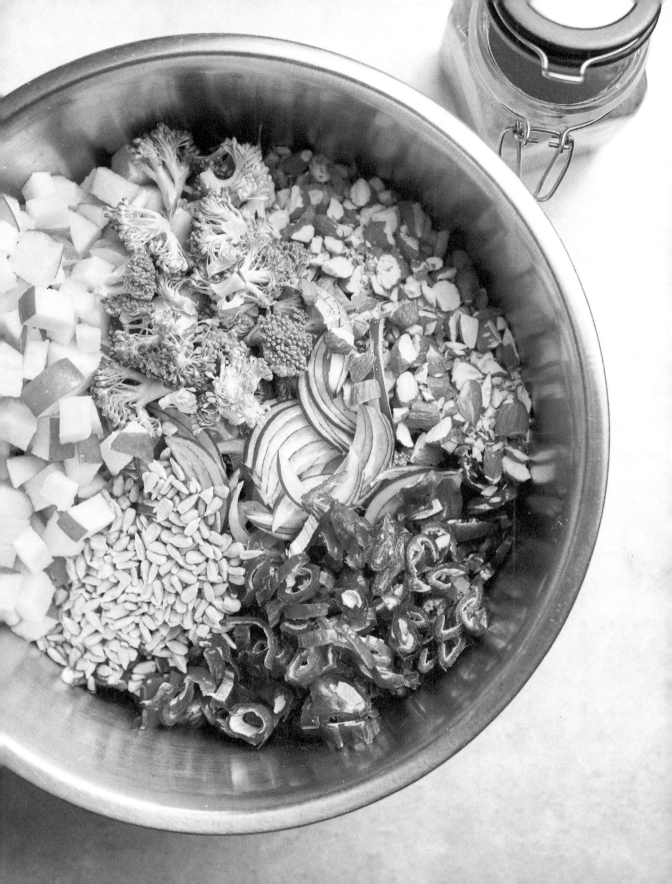

the dirty dozen™ and the clean fifteen™

A nonprofit environmental watchdog organization called Environmental Working Group (EWG) looks at data supplied by the U.S. Department of Agriculture (USDA) and the Food and Drug Administration (FDA) about pesticide residues. Each year it compiles a list of the best and worst pesticide loads found in commercial crops. You can use these lists to decide which fruits and vegetables to buy organic to minimize your exposure to pesticides and which produce is considered safe enough to buy conventionally. This does not mean they are pesticide-free, though, so wash these and all fruits and vegetables thoroughly.

DIRTY DOZEN

Apples	Peaches
Bell peppers	Pears
Celery	Potatoes
Cherries	Spinach
Grapes	Strawberries
Nectarines	Tomatoes

CLEAN FIFTEEN

Asparagus	Kiwis
Avocados	Mangos
Cabbage	Onions
Cantaloupe (domestic)	Papayas
Cauliflower	Pineapples
Eggplant	Sweet corn
Grapefruit	Sweet peas (frozen)
Honeydew melon	

measurement conversions

VOLUME EQUIVALENTS (LIQUID)		
US Standard (ounces)	US Standard (approximate)	Metric
2 tablespoons	1 fl. oz.	30 mL
¼ cup	2 fl. oz.	60 mL
½ cup	4 fl. oz.	120 mL
1 cup	8 fl. oz.	240 mL
1½ cups	12 fl. oz	355 mL
2 cups or 1 pint	16 fl. oz.	475 mL
4 cups or 1 quart	32 fl. oz.	1 L
1 gallon	128 fl. oz.	4 L

OVEN TEMPERATURES	
Fahrenheit (F)	Celsius (C) (approximate)
250°F	120°C
300°F	150°C
325°F	165°C
350°F	180°C
375°F	190°C
400°F	200°C
425°F	220°C
450°F	230°C

VOLUME EQUIVALENTS (DRY)	
US Standard	Metric (approximate)
⅛ teaspoon	0.5 mL
¼ teaspoon	1 mL
½ teaspoon	2 mL
¾ teaspoon	4 mL
1 teaspoon	5 mL
1 tablespoon	15 mL
¼ cup	59 mL
⅓ cup	79 mL
½ cup	118 mL
⅔ cup	156 mL
¾ cup	177 mL
1 cup	235 mL
2 cups or 1 pint	475 mL
3 cups	700 mL
4 cups or 1 quart	1 L

WEIGHT EQUIVALENTS	
US Standard	Metric (approximate)
½ ounce	15 g
1 ounce	30 g
2 ounces	60 g
4 ounces	115 g
8 ounces	225 g
12 ounces	340 g
16 ounces or 1 pound	455 g

resources

When looking to improve your lifestyle and well-being, it is always good to have a supply of trusted materials and resources to help guide your efforts. The following are resources that I find insightful, useful, and motivating in my efforts to stay on top of the trends and knowledge needed for my personal wellness journey.

Dr. Andrew Weil is a physician and guru of anti-inflammatory wellness. The advice in his books and on his website, pairs science-based evidence with an alternative and holistic integrative medicine approach. I agree most with Dr. Weil's message that each body is different, so each person needs to find a personalized version of health. *www.drweil.com*

Epicurious is a cooking resource that even the least kitchen-savvy individual can find helpful. From simple how-to instructions to reviews on kitchen appliances and seasonal recipes, this site has it all. While it isn't necessarily focused on plant-based eating, there are plenty of recipes lacking animal products to choose from. *www.epicurious.com*

Forks Over Knives is a health-promoting, plant-based meal planning, and recipe-sharing community. If you are in need of motivating, real-life success stories from others who have improved their health by eating a plant-based diet, this resource is for you. *www.forksoverknives.com*

Healthyish from *Bon Appetit* is a modern look at what it means to be healthy. The digital resource showcases current trends in the food world, especially those that focus on lifestyle and wellness principles. The recipes are not your boring version of healthy meals. While not all plant based, they do focus on minimalism and using whole, simple ingredients to create vibrant, balanced meals. If you're looking to break out of the brown rice and tofu rut, this will become your go-to source of food inspiration. *www.bonappetit.com/healthyish*

Michael Pollan is a Harvard lecturer who is well known for his writing on the culture of food consumption. Reading his books, specifically *In Defense of Food* and *The Omnivore's Dilemma*, may help and inspire you if you've been struggling with your eating habits or want to better understand what to eat and why. *www.michaelpollan.com*

Well+Good is a website and social media presence that provides inspiration on all topics wellness, including recipes, nutrition, fitness, style, travel, and relationships. The bright photography and diverse posts from contributors across the globe will help you understand there are many forms of wellness and ways to incorporate more of the practices into your own lifestyle. *www.wellandgood.com*

references

Boeing, Heiner, Angela Bechthold, Achim Bub, Sabine Ellinger, Dirk Haller, Anja Kroke, Eva
  Leschik-Bonnet, Manfred J. Müller, Helmut Oberritter, Matthias Schulze, Peter Stehle,
  and Bernhard Watzl. "Critical Review: Vegetables and Fruit in the Prevention of Chronic
  Diseases." *European Journal of Nutrition* 51, no. 6 (2012): 637–63. doi:10.1007
  /s00394-012-0380-y.

Boseley, Sarah. "Low-Calorie Diet Offers Hope of Cure for Type 2 Diabetes." *The Guardian.*
  Accessed June 2018. www.theguardian.com/society/2011/jun/24/low-calorie-diet
  -hope-cure-diabetes.

Bray, George A., and Barry M. Popkin. "Dietary Sugar and Body Weight: Have We Reached a
  Crisis in the Epidemic of Obesity and Diabetes?" *Diabetes Care* 37, no. 4 (2014): 950–56.
  doi:10.2337/dc13-2085.

Diguilo, S. NBC News. "How What You Eat Affects How You Sleep." Accessed July 2018.
  www.nbcnews.com/better/health/how-what-you-eat-affects-how-you-sleep-ncna805256.

Gallagher, James. "Processed Meats Do Cause Cancer—WHO." *BBC News.* Accessed August
  2018. www.bbc.com/news/health-34615621.

Jung, Hana, C.-Y. Oliver Chen, Jeffrey B. Blumberg, and Ho-Kyung Kwak. "The Effect of
  Almonds on Vitamin E Status and Cardiovascular Risk Factors in Korean Adults: A
  Randomized Clinical Trial." *European Journal of Nutrition* 57, no. 6 (2017): 2069–079.
  doi:10.1007/s00394-017-1480-5.

Lally, Phillippa, Cornelia H. M. Van Jaarsveld, Henry W. W. Potts, and Jane Wardle. "How Are
  Habits Formed: Modelling Habit Formation in the Real World." *European Journal of Social
  Psychology* 40, no. 6 (2009): 998–1009. doi:10.1002/ejsp.674.

Leahey, T. "What Are the Best Motivators for Successful and Sustained Weight Loss?"
  US News Health. Accessed August 2018. health.usnews.com/health-news/blogs
  /eat-run/articles/2016-03-10/what-are-the-best-motivators-for-successful-and
  -sustained-weight-loss.

Liu, Y., A. G. Wheaton, D. P. Chapman, and H. Lu. *Morbidity and Mortality Weekly Report.*
  Report. Centers for Disease Control and Prevention. 6th ed. Vol. 65. 136–41. Accessed
  August 2018. www.cdc.gov/mmwr/volumes/65/wr/pdfs/mm6506.pdf.

Nichols, Hannah. "The Top 10 Leading Causes of Death in the United States." *Medical News
  Today.* Accessed August 2018. www.medicalnewstoday.com/articles/282929.php.

Oaklander, M. "Why Organic Food Might Be Worth the High Price." *TIME Health*. February 2016. www.time.com/4206738/organic-food-worth-the-price-study.

"Overweight & Obesity." Centers for Disease Control and Prevention. August 13, 2018. Accessed August 2018. www.cdc.gov/obesity/data/adult.html.

Produce for Better Health Foundation. "State of the Plate, 2015 Study on America's Consumption of Fruit and Vegetables." Accessed June 2018. www.pbhfoundation.org/pdfs/about/res/pbh_res/State_of_the_Plate_2015_WEB_Bookmarked.pdf.

Rockin' Health (blog). "How I Overcame Depression by Changing My Diet." Accessed June 2018. www.leannebrunelle.com/overcame-depression-changing-diet.

Sifferlin, A. "The Weight Loss Trap: Why Your Diet Isn't Working." *TIME Health*. Accessed August 2018. www.time.com/collection/guide-to-weight-loss/4793832/the-weight-loss-trap.

Slavin, J. L., and B. Lloyd. "Health Benefits of Fruits and Vegetables." *Advanced Nutrition* 3, no. 4 (July 2012): 506–516.

Steele, Euridice Martínez, Barry M. Popkin, Boyd Swinburn, and Carlos A. Monteiro. "The Share of Ultra-processed Foods and the Overall Nutritional Quality of Diets in the US: Evidence from a Nationally Representative Cross-sectional Study." *Population Health Metrics* 15, no. 1 (2017). doi:10.1186/s12963-017-0119-3.

Tuso, Philip. "Nutritional Update for Physicians: Plant-Based Diets." *The Permanente Journal* 17, no. 2 (2013): 61–66. doi:10.7812/tpp/12-085.

World Health Organization. "Unhealthy Diet as a Risk Factor for Chronic Disease." Accessed August 2018. www.who.int/ncds/surveillance/steps/resources/unhealthy_diet_rationale.pdf.

Wu, Yanling, Yanping Ding, Yoshimasa Tanaka, and Wen Zhang. "Risk Factors Contributing to Type 2 Diabetes and Recent Advances in the Treatment and Prevention." *International Journal of Medical Sciences* 11, no. 11 (2014): 1185–200. doi:10.7150/ijms.10001.

recipe index

index

acknowledgments

This book was written with support and inspiration from those around me. Most notably my parents, Rick and Janet, inspired me to have an adventurous relationship with food throughout my life. I was lucky to be exposed to everything from escargot and microwavable rice bowls to veggie burgers and homemade meatloaf, without pressure to gravitate toward one or the other. I'm most thankful for the baked cheese and chocolate chip sandwiches my father made on the rare night he was in charge of dinner and the biscuits my mom baked that were so hard we used them as Frisbees in the yard. Without these fond kitchen attempts from my folks, I might never have tried so hard to explore food and learn to cook for myself.

A huge thank-you is also owed to Luke Russell, who continues to support my trials in the kitchen, sink full of dishes, and pestering to sample a new recipe. He is responsible for refining my healthy recipe creativity, resulting in more approachable techniques and accessible ingredients without compromising on taste.

I'd also like to thank my entire audience of clients and social followers who provide inspiration to showcase an authentic approach to living a healthy, well-balanced life.

about the author

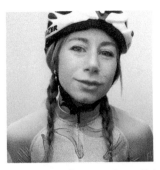

Lori Nedescu, MS, RD, CSSD, is a self-taught personal chef and qualified board-certified sports dietitian–nutritionist. She holds a master's degree in human nutrition and has racked up over 11 years of professional experience in the dynamic field of wellness in roles including recipe demonstrator, corporate wellness coach, public speaker, digital media producer, personal nutrition advisor, and freelance author. As an elite road cyclist and marathon runner who was diagnosed with celiac disease, Lori understands firsthand that eating a nutritious, whole foods diet can greatly affect one's performance, mood, and health and overall increase quality of life. Through her brand, The Cadence Kitchen, Lori provides a fun and authentic approach to food, nutrition, fitness, and lifestyle counseling. Follow her @CadenceKitchen.

NOTES

NOTES

NOTES

NOTES

NOTES

NOTES

NOTES

NOTES

NOTES